PET ER

PET

*Memoirs
of an
Animal Doctor*

ER

George A. Porter

4-12-03

To Jennifer

Enjoy!

George A. Porter

HILLSBORO PRESS

FRANKLIN, TENNESSEE

Printed in the United States of America

03 02 01 00 99   1 2 3 4 5

Library of Congress Catalog Card Number: 99-61912

ISBN: 1-57736-149-0

Cover design by Gary Bozeman

Published by
HILLSBORO PRESS
an imprint of
PROVIDENCE HOUSE PUBLISHERS
238 Seaboard Lane • Franklin, Tennessee 37067
800-321-5692
www.providencehouse.com

Pet ER *is dedicated to my loving wife, Marilyn,
who has stood by my side and supported me
in the many decisions of life. Marilyn's effort
in almost single-handedly raising our three sons
in a Christian environment while I was
mostly unavailable, speaks well of her desire
to be a model mother and wife.
Marilyn's Christian influence has affected
the entire family and permeated all that have
come in contact with her.*

*To Marilyn, alone, I owe what success I have
achieved during my life span.*

CONTENTS

ACKNOWLEDGMENTS

First of all, I want to thank my wife, Marilyn, for inspiring me to write down some of my experiences in veterinary emergency medicine and then putting up with me many days while I endeavored to put it into legible print.

I also have many thanks to extend to my sons, Bradley, Bartell, and James, who helped me to recall cases that had, for the time being, escaped my memory.

Bradley and James introduced me to the computer world and assisted me through the frustrations of learning a language I had never heard of before. They then trained me to be proficient enough to compose on my Imac.

I wish to thank my daughters-in-law, Leslie and Lorraine, for the time they spent editing for spelling, grammar, and sentence structure, and my colleague, Teresa Benton, for editing *Pet ER* from the medical perspective.

Most of all, I owe the subject matter in this book to my clients and their pets, my patients, for without the exciting and sometimes frustrating emergencies that occurred on their part, I would not have the material to write about.

PET *ER* contains stories that have occurred in my practice of veterinary emergency medicine. It also includes the involvement with my family. My wife, Marilyn (Marna), and my three sons, Bradley (Allen), Bartell (George), and James (Albert), all were significantly involved in my professional life. My family's participation was not necessarily associated with the specific cases I wrote about nor were these cases written in any specific sequence.

I graduated from the University of California at Davis in 1962 and commenced my practice career in Torrance, California, in the field of small animal medicine. After five years as an associate, it was time for me to move on. I contracted with six different hospitals to work a specific day a week for them. Since I was involved with these hospitals, I agreed to take all of their night, weekend, and holiday emergencies. Being available for these six hospitals encouraged me to get involved with five more. Now I was covering for eleven hospitals for their off-hour emergencies.

I found it necessary to adjust to a new lifestyle—that of being available. I frequently slept in short stretches, and I was constantly within telephone range. Marilyn became my answering service as she forwarded the incoming messages from the four answering services that received calls from the eleven hospitals.

In 1970 I opened my own practice in Redondo Beach. I stopped working at other hospitals during the day, but I continued to take emergencies for the eleven hospitals—plus my own—which now made twelve. All the emergencies were taken at the referring hospital and that involved considerable time on the road.

I was accustomed to using a gas anesthetic machine at school and was disappointed when I got involved in private practice for few hospitals owned them. They were still using intravenous long-acting anesthetics. To make my emergency life easier, I purchased a Heidbrink gas machine with a metafane vaporizor. In order to have it with me all the time, I modified the trunk of my Mustang and installed styrofoam sections to hold the various parts when I disassembled the machine. The lives of my patients now became much easier for me to manage and much safer for my surgery cases.

Immediately I became very busy. I was available for emergencies for six years—from 1967 until 1974. During this period of time, I logged an average of over one hundred emergencies each month.

At a veterinary symposium, I was privileged to meet James Herriot. In the course of our conversation I had the opportunity to relate several of my experiences in emergency medicine. He suggested that I should jot some of them down. Following his advice, I was inspired to compile numerous events and thus the genesis of PET ER.

PETER

ER

1

HAM BONE

My last patient of the day had been treated and the owner had just exited the examination room with her cat Chaucer snuggled in her arms. I gave a sigh of relief. It had been a long and strenuous day and was now past normal closing time. I was glad that I would soon be heading for home, for fog was creeping in from the ocean and gradually surrounding the city in its silent grasp. This confirmed the weatherman's prediction that the South Bay would be fogbound before morning. My chances of having to respond to a night emergency were minimal, for my clients would not want to struggle through the fog any more than I.

After a cautious drive home, it felt good to finally pull into our driveway. Marna was standing at the kitchen window and probably preparing our evening meal. All I could think about was a good hot home-cooked meal, and then time afterwards to romp with our three sons in the family room in front of the fireplace.

I entered the kitchen and immediately noticed a thermos and a brown bag on the kitchen counter. This was not a good sign. My evening plans had changed. Marna had intercepted a call from the answering service that requested my presence at the Manhattan Beach hospital. I checked in with the service in order to learn more about the nature of the emergency. Doing this enabled me to be better prepared in handling the specifics of any particular case. The patient I was about to see had a bone lodged in its mouth and had been frantically attempting to get it out, but to no avail.

My coat and tie were shed and I donned a sweater. I ruffled up Albert's hair, gave Marna a peck on the cheek, and gave each of the boys a high five and hugs before exiting the house. My sack dinner and coffee were in the seat beside me as I headed west, then north up the coast to my evening's destination. The fog had indeed become dense, and driving was more of a hazard then when I had originally driven home. Ironically, I passed the hospital where I had practiced during the day. I realized that if the call had come in a little sooner I would not have had to double back on this trip to Manhattan Beach. It took me ten to fifteen minutes longer than normal to reach my destination because of the fog and the slow cautious drivers who were also out on the road.

As I pulled into the parking lot, the evening's client pulled in right behind me. In his arms was a red dachschund. Inside I was introduced more formally to Oso, an oh-so small miniature doxie. Oso was tossing her head from side to side in a frantic manner and in doing this was slinging saliva everywhere. We got her into the hospital and up on the exam table. Oso had a bone, a very special bone, in her mouth. This bone was a ring bone from a slice of ham. The Baxters had given it to Oso and she had enjoyed chewing on it, but in the process the grease from the marrow of the ham and her saliva had united to lubricate the bone in such a manner that it became slippery. The bone was then able to slide over her lower canine teeth and become firmly lodged around her mandible. Oso was badly frightened as she could not swallow with this structure in her mouth, and I suspected that she had the feeling she was about to drown in her own saliva.

Mr. Baxter accompanied me as I took Oso into the treatment room. He was an able assistant, for he held Oso securely as I administered a short-acting surital anesthetic intravenously. As the surital entered Oso's bloodstream, she gradually relaxed in Mr. Baxter's arms. Gently he laid her upon a towel on the treatment table. In the meantime I had located the necessary instrument that was needed to remove the ring bone from her lower jaw. Finally Oso was sufficiently relaxed for me to proceed. A tooth splitter was slipped in between her mandible and the bone. Pressure was applied and the bone was severed. The separated halves of the bone flew across the room. Her mandible was badly abraded by the bone. The likelihood that she had pawed at the bone in an attempt to remove it from its secure position was logical. The abraded area was bleeding and rather swollen. Some furacin ointment was rubbed into the lesion but I knew that it would not last there long, for as soon as she woke up, she would lick it off. In animals it is necessary to use topical medications which cause no harm to the pet via the digestive system because if they can reach the location with their tongue, they will attempt to lick it off. Injections of both penicillin and vetalog, a steroid, were given to counter the swelling and reduce the possibility of infection. Oso was temporarily placed upon a towel in the recovery ward cage while the anesthetic wore off, and I began taking care of the business end of the night's emergency.

The pieces of bone were picked up and taken out front and shown to Mrs. Baxter. Both of the Baxters were amazed that such a small bone they had given their pet to enjoy had caused such a problem.

My patient was beginning to wake up so I hurriedly finished the business portion of the evening before returning to the recovery room and bringing Oso out to the Baxters. Oso was still slightly groggy, but I assured the Baxters that the effect of the anesthetic would soon wear off and that she would probably be running around the house before long. There was no need to caution the Baxters about being careful in the future, for the episode spoke for itself.

After the Baxters departed, I proceeded to clean up the examination room, the treatment room, and the cage that Oso had occupied. I turned off the lights and was locking the front door when Mr. Baxter appeared and I wondered what had gone wrong.

He reassured me that all was well but that he would like to have the bone that had been removed. He wanted to give it to his daughter to take to school for show-and-tell. I returned to the hospital and fished the bone out of the trash and presented it to Mr. Baxter. We had a good laugh about the evening's event and he headed for home with his trophy.

As I was locking the door again, the phone rang. I returned to the reception desk and answered the call on the hospital's back line. It was Marna. Another call had come in. This time it was close by in Hawthorne. I checked in with the answering service that had relayed the call and found that the Johnsons were on the way to the Hawthorne hospital with a dog having convulsions. I was on my way again on that foggy evening.

The Johnsons were waiting for me when I arrived. Their dog was wrapped in a blanket and held closely by Mrs. Johnson. Mr. Johnson carried a basket. As I was unlocking the front door, I introduced myself to the couple and they in turn introduced me to Topsy, their female Llasso Apso. In the basket were four puppies about ten days old that were squirming and making puppy sounds.

Topsy was examined and my suspicions were confirmed. I diagnosed her with eclampsia. Eclampsia is a condition in a lactating bitch involving a loss of calcium in the bloodstream called hypocalcemia. She was producing milk faster than the vascular system can recover calcium from the body. In a lactating mother the demand for calcium has priority. She needed to have an intravenous drip of a calcium solution. The Johnsons helped to hold her still for a moment while I established an IV drip. It was to be a slow drip so the tubing was taped to her leg. When the rate of one drop of solution every four seconds was established, I put the recumbent Topsy in an observation cage with all of the attached apparatus.

Returning to the exam room, I explained to the Johnsons that we would have to wait for awhile while the solution was being pumped into Topsy's system. I made three cups of coffee and returned to the front of the hospital and sat down with the couple for a little conversation. Mr. Johnson had been raised on a farm and we got into a discussion comparing bovine milk fever and eclampsia. Topsy was checked intermittently and she was gradually showing improvement as the tremors were not as evident. She was even trying to regain her footing.

I explained to the Johnsons that this condition could recur and that it would be necessary for them to feed the pups by hand during the day and then to let the pups nurse during the night. They were delighted about these instructions, for it meant that they would not have to get up and bottle-feed the four pups two or more times during the night.

Topsy was disconnected from the IV. The Johnsons were given some puppy formula as well as some pet nursing bottles. Careful instructions were given to keep Topsy away from her puppies during the daylight hours because if excess lactation occurred, Topsy could be susceptible to more convulsions. It was somewhat difficult to explain that milk is not produced in any quantity when the pressure is high in the breasts. However, if the pressure is relieved rapidly, as in nursing, a large quantity of milk is rapidly produced which is a precursor to a possible repetition of the symptoms. The couple, after asking several questions, appeared to be satisfied with both my explanation and instructions. They left and I sat down for another cup of coffee and ate my meat loaf sandwich that Marna had fixed. Then I cleaned up the hospital, locked up the premises, and headed for home.

The fog appeared to have thickened slightly. The traffic was sparse. Marna was still up when I pulled into the driveway but I knew that the boys would be fast asleep, for by now the hour hand of the clock was pushing twelve. Slipping into the boys' rooms, I gave each of them a good-night kiss and silently promised them I would see them at breakfast. I was still bright-eyed and bushy-tailed. Marna was sleepy but she still fixed decaf coffee and we sat down for a few moments to share our day's activities. Marna had assumed my responsibility of reading a bedtime story to the boys. She had become so engrossed in the book that she had not noticed that all three were sound asleep. She thought that the boys might have been bored. Marna claimed that I was much more animated when I read stories and that helped keep the boys awake.

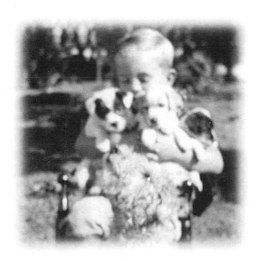

2

CAT IN THE DRYER

It was a pleasant evening. Dinner was over and the dishes were done. Marna, the boys, and I were out on the patio enjoying our time together. Marna had made some popcorn and each of us had our own supply. We were amused watching the boys protect their shares from Greta, our German shorthaired pointer, who was constantly begging for a handout. The moon was just breaking the edge of the horizon. It was so calm and blissful—it was until the phone rang.

Marna answered the phone and then referred the call to me. It was the answering service. They needed help. The lady calling the hospital emergency line was frantic. No information could be obtained. I asked to be connected and the only sound over the receiver was, "Toby is dying, Toby is dying!" I could not calm her down nor could I get any information from her either. The service had told me from which hospital she had called. Finally I said, "Please listen carefully to me. Do you know where the hospital is located?" She was able to respond. I told her that I would be there in ten minutes and was on my way.

I arrived at the hospital first and was in the exam room when she arrived with Toby. She brought her cat into the exam room immediately and placed him on the table. Toby was wrapped in a towel and was very still. Picking up my stethoscope, I listened to the cat's chest and could only perceive a very weak heartbeat. Toby also was barely breathing. A very swollen tongue blocked her throat. Something had to be done right now or she would certainly suffocate.

At this point in the proceedings, the owner announced, "I am going out to the other room. I don't want to watch Toby die." Toby's tongue was blue in color and so swollen that it protruded from her mouth. It was utterly impossible to even consider passing a tracheal tube. Immediate action on my part was essential. I grabbed a scalpel and made a ventral incision in Toby's neck, exposing the trachea. Another incision was made between the trachea rings and a small tube was inserted between the rings. Finally Toby inhaled a breath of fresh air. Her chest expanded and I gave a sigh of relief. The skin on Toby's neck was grasped—it felt like dry leather. It would not spring back into place as it should. This indicated to me that she was badly dehydrated. It was easy to establish an IV tube as my patient was still motionless, and I began to administer saline solution directly into her vein. Solu-delta-cortef solution was injected directly into the IV tube for a quick antishock treatment. Ever so slowly Toby was showing signs of coming back into this world. She was responding to the blink reflex when I touched her eyelids and was commencing to knead her paws. These were encouraging signs.

Toby was caged with the IV tube in place and the solution was reduced to one drop every six seconds. I watched her carefully for ten minutes or so to be certain that her progress continued. Finally her condition was stable. Curiosity got the better of me so I returned to the front room to learn more about the case I was treating. The lady in the reception room did have a name, Hoeltke. She explained to me what had apparently happened.

Case histories are very helpful as well as interesting and I listened intently as she related the anamnesis to me. "I had taken some clothes out of the clothes dryer and thoughtlessly left the dryer door open. Toby had climbed into the dryer to take a nap on the remaining warm clothes. One of my children had come by, saw the dryer door open with clothes still in it, shut the dryer door, and started it up again. Possibly ten to twenty minutes later, Tim came by the dryer and heard bumping sounds. Tim asked me whose shoes had been washed and were now being dried. The question did not sink in for a couple of minutes and I suddenly realized that no shoes should be in the dryer. I rushed into the laundry room, opened the dryer door, and there was Toby in a comatose state."

The problem now was to get Toby back to her normal state. Her tongue had been bitten many times as she tumbled about in the dryer. It had swollen to such a degree that she was unable to keep it in her mouth.

I washed the tongue with water and squirted as much water as possible into her mouth. The IV drip was carefully monitored. That faraway look in her eyes was disappearing and she began flexing her paws more. Her heart rate was becoming stronger and her respiration was improving as well.

Mrs. Hoeltke and I kept a vigil for over an hour and then I advised her that she might as well return home and report to her family that Toby had not died. Toby would be monitored intermittently throughout the night, and in the morning I would turn over the responsibility of her care to the doctor in charge of the hospital.

Toby was checked for the last time about three in the morning and her condition was stable. She even tried to purr when I petted her. Toby remained in the hospital for four days until the trachea tube could be removed and the neck sutured.

It was about two months later when I ran into Mrs. Hoeltke at the grocery store. Toby was doing fine. Her tongue had remained black and blue for almost a week and then it had turned a ghastly yellow before it reverted to its normal pink color. Toby had to be fed a very soft diet as well as water with a syringe for a period of time because she could not lap up anything. Toby now appeared fine and was eating well. Mrs. Hoeltke made me chuckle when she told me that Toby would come into the house only by way of the front door. She would not enter through the back door that opened into the utility room and contained the dryer.

3

Two Boys and a Dog

It was still early in the evening when a call came in to go to the Lawndale hospital. A Mrs. Williams agreed to meet me at the hospital with her dog that had a badly swollen muzzle. We both reached the hospital at about the same time. Mrs. Williams had her two sons with her. Jack was, I guess, about five years old and John was about three. Their dog, Cinder, a four-year-old black Labrador had a very swollen cheek. Jack held him on a leash.

Cinder had been playing in the backyard with the boys. All of a sudden Cinder gave a yelp and frantically began rubbing the side of her face against the grass. This had happened about an hour ago and now her face was very swollen on the left side. I surmised that she had been bitten by an insect.

I picked up Cinder and placed her on the exam table. Mrs. Williams was asked to hold her and she dutifully replied that she would. At this moment, Jack opened a drawer behind me—so far, in fact, that all of the contents of the drawer became scattered around the room. Needles and syringes lay in disarray over the floor. Mrs. Williams started shouting at Jack about his misbehavior. She was so intent on reprimanding Jack that she negligently released her grip on Cinder. Cinder, now unfettered, jumped off the table and made a beeline for her port of entry, the reception room. Mrs. Williams was very apologetic and commenced to help me pick up the articles that decorated the floor. Mrs. Williams and I were

11

interrupted by John who announced that Cinder had "pooped" on the floor in the front room.

I thought it would be more prudent to abandon picking up the syringes and needles and clean up the dog mess before one of the boys stepped in it. I was too late. John had already stepped in it and was tracking it around the front of the hospital. Mrs. Williams became unglued. She started screaming at Jack to hold still. Her loud voice panicked Cinder who started running around dragging the leash that was still attached to her collar through the excretion on the floor. We attempted to corner Cinder by trying to grab her or the leash. Cinder must have thought it was some sort of a game. In any event, during the excitement, she managed to step into the original mess as well as the mess being tracked around by John.

Order was finally restored. Cinder was again placed up on the exam table and this time held even more securely by Mrs. Williams. Jack and John were rooted in chairs in the front room and ordered to remain there by their mother. A very pronounced odor of animal waste prevailed.

I gave my four-footed friend an antihistamine injection of benedryl to alleviate her swollen face. After I washed all four feet, I carried her via a very circuitous route to the front door and placed her into the Williamses' automobile. The boys had followed the explicit instructions of their mother and had remained glued to their chairs in the reception room. My next job was to remove each of the boys' shoes and scrub the shoes in the tub until clean rather than try to clean them while the boys were wearing them. The boys were properly reshod and individually carried out to the car to join Cinder. Mrs. Williams again apologized while we were completing the business portion of the evening's misfortune. She then also took a careful route to the front door.

Returning to the hospital, I picked up the remaining syringes and needles which hid in various nooks and crannies. I changed into my janitorial shoes and smock before attacking the floor and the canine decorations that still lay on it. After the floor was thoroughly mopped, the only evidence of the disaster was a lingering odor that still prevailed. This clean-up effort was absolutely necessary, for I knew that I would not like to be the person to open the front door of any facility and see and smell the mess that had been present.

Heading for home, I pondered as to how I could have handled this emergency differently. I decided that because of the confusion and the speed with which it happened I should be thankful that I was away from home for only three hours. I did learn that excitable dogs and uncontrollable children combined with a frantic parent can add a lot of stress to any emergency.

It was about bedtime when I got my next call. This call was from Manhattan Beach and it was about a cat that had been rescued from an oil sump, a reservoir that holds waste oil. I had never heard of a cat surviving such an experience—usually they inhale some of the fluid and then succumb because of respiratory problems.

Some "good Samaritans" brought in this cat in a plastic garbage bag with only its head sticking out. I took the cat, bag and all, and dumped the whole package into a cage. They left the required deposit and I obtained the necessary name, address, and telephone number. I was to call them later in the evening and give them a progress report.

The entire bag was placed in the bathtub. Since the cat's head was exposed, I put a restraining leash around its neck and then carefully removed the bag in the hopes of restricting the black and gooey contents to the tub area. No sooner was the bag removed that the cat shook itself. At this point, I realized that I had used poor judgment. Black, oily sludge was everywhere—on the walls, ceiling, floor, and anything else within twelve feet of the tub. I stood there for a few moments with my hands on my hips and surveyed the scene in disgust.

It took six latherings with Amway's detergent soap, LOC, to cut the oil. With each application of soap I was getting a better glimpse of my patient. It wasn't a black cat at all but a beautiful blue-point Siamese with beet-red skin due to the irritation of the oil sludge and the detergent. A local pharmacy was called and the pharmacist recommended a shampoo that would soothe the skin. I then administered a steroid injection of azium to help reduce the skin inflammation. I put the wet Siamese into a holding cage, and then drove to the pharmacy to pick up the aforementioned shampoo.

Kitty was not a happy camper about getting into the bathtub again. She received two more thorough latherings, and then after the second application, she was left for almost twenty minutes in the tub while the medication in the shampoo soaked into her skin and soothed the irritation. After I toweled her and placed her into a dryer cage, I began the cleanup. I looked around the hospital and located a step stool in order to help me reach the oil spots on the walls and ceiling. It took a little over an hour to remove all of that black tarry substance.

Now it was time to call the people who had brought in the cat and give them the promised progress report. When informed that Kitty was all cleaned up and doing well, they asked me what she looked like. Kitty's features were described and the Samaritans said, "Oh, that's Showboat, and she belongs to a neighbor down the street." They agreed to call Showboat's owners and tell them where their cat was. No one answered the phone so they walked down the street to talk to their neighbors in person.

While there a young boy who lived in the area came around the house and asked them if they had seen Showboat. The Samaritans told the boy that the cat had been rescued from an oil sump and that it was now being cared for at the hospital. The young man had been house-sitting Showboat while the owners were out of town. It is likely that Showboat had escaped from the garage at feeding time without the young man being aware of it. When he went to feed Showboat that evening, the cat food remained untouched in the food dish and he could not find the cat anywhere in the garage. Why the cat found refuge in the area of the oil sump is open for speculation, but it is likely that some dog may have chased Showboat into the oil sump.

As I drove home, I could not help but think about the hours I had spent cleaning cages, tables, tub, walls, and floors. Hopefully, Marna would never be aware of the valuable janitorial skills that I had developed.

4

PUPPIES GALORE

Sunday mornings provided a different routine for me. On occasion I often had as many as six hospitals at which I was responsible for morning treatments. This particular morning only three hospitals required my presence. I awakened early, grabbed a cup of coffee, and headed for my first location of the day. All went well, and after my rounds were completed, I was homeward bound.

Since I started early and finished early that day, I was able to take my family to church, which was a rare occasion. We drove to church in two cars in case I was suddenly called away, and the boys argued over which car they wanted to be in. After we settled their childish disputes, we were on our way.

When we arrived at church, I called the four answering services and gave them the phone number where I could be reached while Marna took the boys to their Sunday school classes. The ushers showed me to a seat that would make an unexpected exit easy for me.

For the first time in awhile, I was able to attend the entire service. This time Allen drove home with me and Marna chauffeured the younger two. We were sitting down at brunch when the phone rang. There was a whelping case that needed attention at the Hawthorne hospital. Allen wanted to go with me. It was often necessary to have an experienced assistant in this type of case and Allen was qualified—he had assisted me several times before in cesarean deliveries. His brothers, George and

15

Albert, begged to go along but they were discouraged by Marna after I flashed a disapproving look to her. It just was not practical to have that many children underfoot when concentration was needed in surgery. Allen and I slipped inconspicuously out the back door and headed north to Hawthorne.

The Hartman's bitch had commenced labor sometime during the night. When the Hartmans found Tina in the morning, she had delivered one dead puppy and was restless. It was evident to them that she had more pups to deliver so they had called the emergency service.

They had made a good decision—Tina was still heavy with pups. I could palpate two and it was likely that even more were present. Tina was so fatigued that she was unable to respond to a hormone injection of oxytocin given to cause uterine contractions. A cesarean section was imminent. While I prepared for surgery, Allen found a cardboard box. He located some bottles and put hot water in them. The bottles were placed in the box and covered with terry cloth towels to provide indirect warmth to the newborn pups.

Tina was given just enough of an injection of the short-acting anesthetic, surital, to facilitate the passing of an endotrachial tube. She was then connected to the metafane gas anesthetic machine. It is very necessary to administer as small an amount of anesthetic as possible to perform the necessary cesarean, for both venous and gas anesthetics can be carried transplacentally to the feti. If too much is given, the pups are doped-up at delivery time and slow to respond.

Surgery proceeded in the prescribed fashion. A pup would be delivered into the world and handed to Allen. He would then clear its throat and get it breathing properly. Then the new arrival would be taken out into the front room and given to the owners to towel off. When dried thoroughly, the pup would be placed into the box on the warm towels. This scenario was repeated three more times for a total of four puppies.

Surgery had been completed and my surgical gloves were being removed when the phone rang. Allen answered it. The service asked Allen to tell me that another whelping case was coming into this hospital. Allen said, "Dad, they're back-to-back today." Knowing that there was a possibility that I might need to use the cesarean pack again today, we cleaned the instruments and put the pack into the autoclave for sterilization. When this task was completed and I was out of the way, Allen cleaned up the surgery room. The Hartmans had followed Allen's instructions; the pups were dry and warm and exhibiting signs that they were hungry.

Allen had prepared the recovery cage and had taken Tina into her reserved cage. By this time my cursory check of the pups was completed and Tina was beginning to stir. The pups were then placed with their mother and as if by magic, they knew exactly what to do. Soon all four pups were nursing and kneading their paws against their mother's breasts, giving the impression they were pumping milk out by their actions. We waited for a few minutes and noting that all was going well, I brought Tina out to the Hartmans and Allen carried the four new arrivals out in the box. Allen and I marveled that, as a team, we were able to bring four healthy pups into the world.

The Hartmans were instructed to call in the morning and give the hospital a current report on Tina and her family and also to make an appointment to have Tina's stitches removed. Tina was not a breed that customarily required the pups' tails to be docked but I did suggest that it might be prudent to consider having the dewclaws surgically removed. It was suggested that they discuss it with the doctor in the morning when they called.

The Isleys arrived with their female terrier, Babe. The Hartman scenario was repeated. This time six healthy pups were introduced into the world by caesarian section. Allen was really gaining experience this afternoon. Babe was not recovering in the desired manner so my recommendation was to keep her and her puppies at the hospital overnight so they could be checked on periodically. The Isleys readily agreed and asked me to call about nine and give them an update.

As we cleaned up the hospital, Allen wondered if I was as hungry as he. We decided that the best way to alleviate hunger was to walk up to the corner hamburger stand and get a sandwich and a soft drink. We loitered there while we indulged and each of us had an ice cream cone to top off our afternoon's efforts. As we sauntered back to the hospital we relived the events of the day. We checked the pups and all were nursing and emitting puppy sounds. The phone rang and the service was asked to cross-connect me to a Mr. Betts. Mr. Betts informed me that their Border collie, Toots, was in difficult labor, a dystocia.

The Bettses were clients of this hospital so we did not have to travel. Thankfully, we had put the surgical pack into the autoclave to sterilize before we had left for our snack. Just as the bell rang indicating that sterilization was complete, the Betts family arrived. Toots was definitely in a troubled labor. Examination revealed that the first pup she was trying to give birth to was in a breech position—it was located across the birth canal. Manually it was possible to change the pup's position to the proper alignment. One hard push from Toots and, behold, I had a newborn pup in my hand. I injected oxytocin intravenously to enable Toots to continue her contractions but she was unable to respond—another caesarean section was necessary. Allen and I again worked as an effective team and soon we were able to boast a total of four puppies in the box in the front room. When Toots was sufficiently awake, we put the pups in the cage with her as we had done before with both Tina and Babe.

Again I felt it was in Toots's best interest to have her and her family remain at the hospital for observation. Now I had two litters to check during the night. Allen helped me to pick up the premises and return everything to its proper location. We then headed home. Allen informed me as we drove along that there was the same number of girl puppies as boy puppies. I was surprised that he had been so observant and I was proud of the assistance that my twelve-year-old son had given me. He had done an outstanding job.

When we arrived home, Allen rushed into the house and told both Marna and his brothers, "Daddy and I delivered puppies back-to-back-to-back." Allen spent considerable time explaining in detail to his younger brothers what he had done. They listened to every detail. Marna and I stood in the doorway and watched Albert and George listening intently. Marna said, "Allen appears to be conducting a seminar."

Several more emergency calls occupied my evening and while I was out, I checked the maternity ward periodically. My last trip was about one-thirty in the morning. I crawled into bed and fell into a deep sleep only to be awakened by that infernal machine invented by Alexander Graham Bell. Fortunately, I have the ability to wake up and be alert enough to answer the telephone before it rings twice. It is also possible for me to conduct a reasonable conversation with the emergency operators as well as the clients they connect me to. After I return from a call, I can put my head on the pillow, and fall asleep quickly. Because of these three factors, I have been able to survive a considerable time as an emergency practitioner.

The answering service had a man on the line who was both rude and obnoxious. She was certain that he had had too much to drink and was calling from some bar. He had repeatedly phoned and was making a nuisance of himself. Her question was, "Would you be willing to talk to him?" I answered, "Yes."

He was definitely drunk. I could also hear bar noises in the background. He asked, "Gosh Doc, I've got a bet going here. If I have my dog cut, would he still jump the back fence?" I responded by saying that if his dog was castrated, it could still jump the back fence but the reasons he may want to jump the fence would be minimized. Before he could ask another question, I thanked him for calling and hung up. I lay awake for a few moments pondering whether he had won or lost the bet.

Monday morning I was up early, for I wanted to check the Hawthorne maternity ward prior to going to work at my scheduled day shift. All the pups were vigorously nursing or sound asleep in a pile. Both bitches were alert and greeted me when the door was opened. It felt good to know that all was well with yesterday's surgeries.

5 —

PEACE OF MIND

Two emergencies had occurred in the early evening. When I returned to the house, it was starting to rain. It was only a drizzle, but the sky looked threatening and I knew that it would only get worse—not better. The boys were not yet in bed so I had the opportunity to tuck them in, hear their prayers, and give them a goodnight hug and kiss. Marna had dinner ready for me by the fireplace and it was nice and cozy that fall evening. Dessert and coffee complemented the evening meal. We sat back to enjoy the fire and another cup of java as we recapped the day's events. I supposed that I would be home the rest of the night, for it had started to rain hard and no one would want to be out in wet weather either.

I commented to Marna how much I was enjoying the fire and coffee as well as the time we were sharing together when the phone rang. Mrs. McVale had a dog that was scratching itself. In questioning her, she explained that her dog was paying a lot of attention to the side of its neck. I recommended that she cut the foot out of a sock and then slip the top part over the dog's head to construct a turtleneck collar. Then I told her to take the toe of the sock and tape it over the foot that was doing the damage. In the morning when her regular veterinarian opened his office she should then see him for a follow-up.

Sitting back in my chair holding a hot cup of coffee in front of the fire, I relished the fact that I would not have to go out in this stormy evening. The phone rang again. It was Mrs. McVale. She had called another hospital and a different answering service was responding. I assured her that the problem was not life threatening and it could be resolved in the morning by her regular veterinarian.

Fifteen minutes later Mrs. McVale was calling through yet a third hospital's exchange. I got the message. She wanted her dog cared for tonight. Her remark was, "Are you the only doctor on duty tonight?" I explained to her that there were several hospitals for which I took emergency cases. We agreed to meet at the first hospital she had called in about half an hour. So much for the stormy evening by the fireplace as well as the steamy cup of coffee. I was on my way.

Mr. and Mrs. McVale arrived on time with their cocker spaniel named Rusty. Rain was now pelting the front window backed by gusts of wind. It was not a night to venture out in, but the McVales were very concerned. I examined Rusty and found that the sock collar was in place and doing an adequate job of protecting the neck. The skin on the neck was inflamed from scratching, but was not abraded. The sock that they had placed on the foot was being held by Mr. McVale. I sort of implied that this emergency could have waited until morning. Mr. McVale looked at his wife and said, "I told you so."

In questioning them a little about Rusty's history, it became evident that Rusty did not have a bed of his own. Rusty slept on their bed with them. Rusty's scratching was annoying them so much that they could not get to sleep. Mrs. McVale was a light sleeper and Rusty's scratching kept her awake. Mr. McVale was a very sound sleeper and nothing bothered him except his wife's continually prodding him to keep the dog from shaking the bed with its scratching. The end result was that neither of them was getting to sleep.

I replaced the stocking on the hind foot and taped it securely with elastic tape. An ampicillin injection to prevent infection and an azium injection to lessen any irritation were given. The McVales were instructed to visit their regular veterinarian when his office opened in the morning.

Mrs. McVale thanked me profusely and gave me a hug before they left. This made me feel a little better about my night out on the town. I have a habit of classifying my cases and this one was filed under the heading of "peace of mind" emergencies. It was likely that now the McVales and their dog would all get a good night of uninterrupted sleep. I headed for home to get mine.

Before the sun peeked over the horizon, I had a call from the Johnsons about Topsy. Topsy was treated two weeks before for eclampsia. We had established a schedule to control the problem. Somehow Topsy had chewed through a partition and managed to get back with her pups. The pups were delighted and had vigorously indulged in this extra feeding from mama. Mama Topsy was also delighted, for the pressure in her breasts had been relieved. We were now back to square one, for Topsy was now exhibiting the same symptoms as before.

Tremors were becoming more intense and more frequent. An intravenous drip was established again and Topsy was assigned to an observation cage. It was now time for me to make some instant coffee, sit down with the Johnsons, and figure out how we could keep this problem from happening again. We now had one advantage—the pups were older.

The Johnsons were very aware that Topsy was unusually sensitive to eclampsia. I recommended that the pups not nurse at all in the future. They could not envision themselves bottle-feeding four pups four to five times a day, so I suggested an alternative. I told them to locate a large cardboard box and find a jelly-roll pan which would fit inside the box. They should then put the pan in the box, fill the pan with formula or milk, and put the pups in the milk-filled pan. The pups would then be wading in milk and if they could not figure out what to do, the Johnsons should push their muzzles down into the milk. The pups would then commence to lick the milk off their faces and would get the idea of licking milk from the pan.

The pup, milk, pan, and box system had always worked for me. The box serves to keep the pups restrained in the milk-filled pan, and keep the floor much cleaner. The only chore the Johnsons had then was to clean off sixteen paws when dinner was over. In about three days the pups would be drinking milk on their own. I told them to feed the litter just before they retired at night. This late feeding might tend to hold the puppies over until morning.

I disconnected Topsy from the IV drip when she had been restored to normality and wished the Johnsons my best. I headed for home to have a cup of Marna's freshly brewed coffee—a welcomed change to the instant coffee I had been drinking all day.

6

FOUR GUYS AND A DOLL

My trip this evening was to Manhattan Beach—the client's dog that had been vomiting for a couple of hours. When I pulled into the hospital parking lot there were four Harley Davidson motorcycles parked there. Four leather-coated men and a "doll" with a Chihuahua in her arms were waiting for me. When the hospital was opened, the entire group proceeded to enter. The men were unshaven and each seemed to exceed me in height by at least six inches. It was an uncomfortable situation; I was very uneasy.

The men were quiet and very polite. The "doll" did most of the talking. Bandit had apparently eaten something bad. The fact that he had dysentery was evident—the aroma permeated the room. Bandit was unsteady on his feet, and looked in one direction and tried to walk in another. He was more than disoriented. His eyes were well dilated and I was very suspicious that he was under the influence of some type of narcotic.

"Was Bandit outside?" I asked. "No," was the response. "Did he get into something in the house?" "I don't think so," responded the lady. By this time I realized they were becoming evasive to the questions I was firing at them. "Do any of you have an idea what may have made Bandit sick?"

Frustration began to creep over me for no direct answer could be elicited from the group. I continued to bombard them with questions that

I felt could be answered but I received no satisfactory answers. They must have felt that they were being grilled by the local constabulary. I continued my interrogation. They began glancing at each other, giving me the impression they expected one of their party to come forward with some useful information. I told them that I would have to know what Bandit might have gotten into so he could be properly treated. A prolonged silence ensued. It must have lasted a full two minutes. Finally the lady said that Bandit might have gotten into some potato chips. At least the group was beginning to communicate with me. "Where were the chips?" I asked. More glances at each other. "On a table," came the response from one of the men. Now I had two people talking to me.

"Let's approach this logically," I said. "We are looking at a very small dog and you claim he got up on a table and ate some potato chips. All of us have eaten potato chips without any ill effects. What else did he get into?" More glances passed between the members of the motorcycle group. At this stage of the inquisition, two of the men went outside for a "smoke." The lady again appeared to be the spokesperson, for she added, "Maybe it was the seasoning on the chips that caused the problem." "What seasoning did you add to the chips?" I blurted out. From the back of the room came the response, "Hell, Meg, tell the Doc there was PCP on the chips. We can't stay here all night." Finally the truth came out.

I told them I would have to call the poison control center and get their advice. They vehemently objected. My next thought was to hospitalize Bandit, but they rejected that suggestion as well. Bandit was treated as efficiently as possible with the medication available at the hospital.

Needless to say, I recommended that they keep these types of products out of the reach of both pets and children. I also admonished them for using such products. The medical record was filled out and presented to them. At this stage they glanced at each other, and I had the feeling that I would not be paid for my efforts this evening.

The two smokers returned to the reception room. Behind them was a local police officer. The officer should have been an actor, for he said, "Saw your light on, Doc, and just stopped by for a cup of coffee." All of a sudden cash appeared on the counter and the account was resolved. The five thanked me and made a hasty retreat with Bandit.

The officer asked if everything was okay. I assured him that all was well. We never did have coffee together. He had seen the motorcycles out front and the lights on in the hospital. He was suspicious and stopped to see if he could assist me in any way. I thanked him for his concern and told him that I was a bit uneasy about the situation. He recommended that it would always be good to call the precinct before I left home if ever I was sensitive about my safety. I explained that I was not always able to evaluate a situation over the phone. When I arrived at the hospital, I might be unable to call.

As I drove home, I thanked the Lord for keeping me safe. I resolved to be more careful in the future and wondered how I could anticipate this kind of situation again.

I related the evening's events to Marna. I did not wish to frighten her but I wanted her input. We decided that in the future, if I was gone for what might seem too long, she would call the hospital. If I answered and could not converse in front of the clients, I would use a prearranged code word. When Marna heard this word, she would call the local law enforcement agency and ask them to drop by the hospital and see if everything was in order.

FAUX PAS

My trip to the hospital this evening allowed me to get acquainted with Mrs. Wilson, her six-year-old daughter, Sallie, and their dog, Barney. Barney was a cute little four-month-old beagle. His problem was that he could not walk on his left rear leg. I checked Barney's heart and about this time, I realized that Sallie was crying. She was upset because her dog was hurt and had to come to the hospital. Realizing the need to comfort her and reassure her that Barney would be taken care of, I picked her up and placed her on the exam table next to Barney. Now she could see what was happening and she could comfort her pet if she wished. (I frequently will put a child up on the exam table and ask him or her to help me with the diagnosis.) The stethoscope was still hanging over my shoulder so I invited her to assist me with the diagnosis by listening to Barney's heart. I adjusted the stethoscope to fit Sallie and the bell was placed on Barney's chest just over his heart. "What do you hear, Sallie?" was my question. "Tachycardia," was her quick response.

I must have looked very surprised to Mrs. Wilson. She clarified Sallie's response by telling me that her father is a cardiologist. Not only was it a big-word response from a little girl, but it was a very accurate response. Most of the time when a pet is on the examination table, the animal has an anxiety complex and a rapid heartbeat occurs.

I examined Barney's leg and found no fracture. The hip was a different story—it was dislocated. My observation was relayed to Mrs. Wilson. She said that Sallie had come into the house crying because Barney yipped as she picked him up. When she put him on the ground, he would not place his leg down. Sallie then told her mother that she had picked Barney up by his left rear leg.

An x-ray was taken to confirm my suspicion of a dislocation of the left hip. I gave Barney an intravenous injection of surital. This injection would relax the muscles and dope him up enough so that he would not feel any pain during surgical correction. The head of the femur was manipulated to relocate it in the pelvic socket. In order to keep the correction in place, I bound the leg to the body. Barney would be a three-legged dog for three to four days before the splint could be removed.

About fifteen minutes later, Barney was alert enough to be discharged. I carried him out to his anxious family. Barney commenced to wag his tail when he saw Sallie. Sallie was now all smiles. She held Barney on her lap for a few minutes while I gave instructions to her mother about Barney's aftercare. Sallie then carefully bundled Barney up and carried him out to the car.

While in the treatment room, I was located by the answering service. I was connected to a client who had an injured pet. Soon I was on my way to my next case in San Pedro. Twenty minutes later I arrived and found the client waiting for me at the front door.

This client was a boater and lived on a sailboat in the harbor. A few weeks before a friend had given her a Siamese kitten. She really didn't want a pet, but rather than offend her friend she accepted the gift. While she was out sailing, her boat encountered a swell that rocked the boat. She lost her balance and stepped back on the kitten, injuring it. Now she wanted me to put it to sleep. It had an obvious fracture of its left front paw and she could not afford to have the fracture repaired. She again admitted that it was not a good idea to have a pet on the boat so she had made the decision to put the kitten to sleep to eliminate any pain and suffering it was now enduring.

We chatted for a few minutes. Realizing that she was strapped for finances, I suggested that if she would sign a release relinquishing owner-ship of the kitten I would fix the leg and try to find a home for it. I explained that the only expense she would incur would be the emergency fee. She readily agreed. Papers were signed and now I had temporary ownership of an injured seal point Siamese kitten. I affixed a temporary splint to the leg and put the kitten in a cage.

The next morning I had a call from the San Pedro hospital wishing to know who owned the kitten. In my haste I had neglected to fill out a cage card with my name on it. I asked to talk to Jeff, the resident veterinarian, and explained the situation to him. A suitable home was needed for an orphan kitten. I asked Jeff if he could assist me in finding a home for this injured feline. Jeff's response was, "We can't keep the kitten here. Why don't you take the responsibility of placing this kitten." I knew Jeff was correct, for I had admitted the kitten to his hospital. Jeff offered his hospital for the corrective surgery and I accepted his offer.

At the end of my day shift, I called the hospital and asked if their surgery room was available that evening. Then I returned to San Pedro and surgically corrected the leg by installing an intramedullary pin. When surgery was completed, a splint was fashioned so that the limb would not rotate. I could not leave the kitten at the hospital, for the kitten had already overextended its welcome. The only thing that could be done on such short notice was to take this little ball of fur home. I was certain that Jeff would approve of this decision—he, in no way, desired to be involved with an ownership problem.

I wrapped the kitten up in a towel and carried him out to the car. When I got home, I showed Marna the little kitten I was holding. I told her that we would keep him for a few days until we could find someone who wanted him. Marna's only comment was, "What do you mean by 'we'?"

My prayer was answered almost immediately, but not the way I had envisioned. The boys and Marna felt that the kitten could take up residence at our house until the bone had healed enough to take the pin out. I was rather hesitant, but was obviously outvoted.

The next task was to find a suitable name for this male kitten. The boys suggested several names for the kitten. In fact, a rather lively discussion ensued as to which of the boys would have the privilege of selecting the name. Marna intervened and stated that she had not been consulted for an opinion. She reminded us that the kitten had a broken foreleg and had been admitted to our household because the owner had used poor judgment by having it on a boat. The kitten's name should be Faux Pas, for it more or less was related to his experience and it did sound like "fore paw."

After residing in our home for almost eight weeks, Faux Pas became a household fixture. He had investigated every nook and cranny he could find. Even his favorite chair had been selected. He originally picked out my chair by the fire but I was able to encourage him to select another. Each member of the family, including myself, doted on him, and Faux Pas was aware of all of this. He was gradually usurping me in becoming master of the premises. He was accepted as a member of the household and enjoyed this status position for over twelve years.

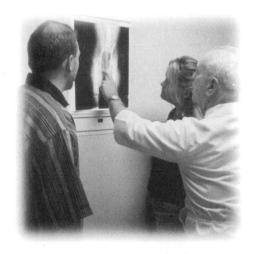

8 —

A SURVIVOR

Bob, a fellow Rotarian, called me just before midnight. Very few calls ever came to me directly. It was the responsibility of the answering service to filter all incoming messages. There was no need for me to inform clients of the time the office opened, to make appointments, or to handle other trivial matters that were the responsibility of the office staffs. My function was to help animals in distress, and all incoming calls were filtered in order to be limited to this purpose only.

Bob knew my home phone number and he called because his sheltie, Ginger, had been in a fight. To be more exact, Ginger had been severely mauled by a pack of dogs. Several dogs in the neighborhood had attacked Ginger that night and this brawl had continued for several minutes. Ginger eventually sought refuge under Bob's bedroom window. At this point, Bob woke up and realized that his dog was in trouble. By the time he dressed and got outside, Ginger was lying on the grass motionless. He checked his dog carefully and realized she was dead. In order to protect her body in the event the pack returned, he got some metal garbage can lids and used them to cover her carcass.

Bob returned to bed but because of this traumatic event he could not get to sleep. He just lay there thinking about Ginger and of all of the pain she must have endured trying to protect herself. Later, he heard the garbage can lids being disturbed. He knew that the dogs had returned and he got up quickly—he intended to teach them a lesson. By the time he got to the garage and found a baseball bat, he had become very emotional about his dog's death. He came around the corner of the house to where Ginger lay. No dogs were in sight. The garbage can lids were moving slightly. Quickly the lids were removed and he then realized that Ginger was breathing. He picked up this pitiful mass of bloody mangled hair, took her into the house, and then called me directly.

We arrived at the Palos Verdes hospital at the same time. He put Ginger on the exam table and I carefully rolled back the blanket to assess the damage. She was comatose and a mess. She was so matted and bloody that it was impossible to ascertain the extent of her injuries. I administered a solution of solu-delta-cortef IV for shock support. While the IV needle was in place, I connected a solution of saline and dextrose and metered it at one drop every three seconds. Both Bob and I monitored her carefully for well over an hour. Her respiration gradually improved and her pulse strengthened. Slowly Ginger's color began to return to normal. Bob had been pacing the floor and muttering to himself. I suggested that he needn't stay at the hospital any longer as there was nothing he could do to help Ginger's condition. He returned home.

As Ginger's pulse continued to improve, blood began to ooze from a multitude of wounds. The actual lesions were difficult to see behind the bloody hair masses. The most critical place appeared to be in her neck where a deep three-inch wound was evident. So I clipped, scrubbed, swabbed with antiseptic, and then went to work. I clamped and ligated the blood vessels. Hair, leaves, grass, and any other foreign matter was removed from the lesion. Finally the wound was closed with sutures.

As I clipped the hair from Ginger's body, more and more lacerations became evident. There were too many puncture wounds to even count and several lacerations as long as two inches. I decided it would be more expedient to clip her entire body. Then I gave her a surgical soap bath. This enabled me to find all of the lesions that needed to be sutured. Next I painted her body with a red zepherine antiseptic and resigned myself to a long surgery. Three hours later I finally backed away from the surgery table. I removed my surgical gloves and turned off the anesthetic machine.

Ginger was monitored in surgery until she started showing eye reflexes. A new bottle of solution was connected to the IV drip system and an antibiotic injection of ampicillin was given in the muscle. Ginger was put into intensive care on a heating pad. I made a full pot of coffee before the huge job of cleaning up the surgery room. When I finished cleaning, I poured a cup of coffee—I knew I would need it, for the night was not over yet for me.

I pulled up a chair in intensive care and drank almost the entire pot of coffee as I watched Ginger's progress. The sun was showing well above the horizon when the regular veterinarian arrived. We discussed my night's case. He had the audacity of accusing me of using a sewing machine on the sheltie! Together we counted twenty-three lesions and over 140 sutures. I headed home, shaved, and reported for my daytime job.

The biggest problem with doing emergency work is that I rarely hear from or see the patient again. I will treat a case at night or on weekends and then turn it over to the home veterinarian for aftercare. I always appreciate a progress report on my cases and infrequently receive one. Progress reports are very important to me because they help me to assess and improve my skills.

Bob's Ginger was a different story. Ginger's progress was unbelievable. Most of her stitches were removed in two weeks—the rest a week later. Every Wednesday at Rotary Club, I received a follow-up report on the case. Ginger's recovery was slow, but this was anticipated since she had been through a severely traumatic experience. Soon, however, she was her old self. Her most profound adjustment was getting used to her nudity immediately after surgery. Apparently she was embarrassed because her beautiful coat had been removed and it took her some time to emotionally adjust.

9

JUST KIDDING

It was a beautiful Saturday evening. The phone had not made a sound all afternoon and my yard work had not been interrupted except for several sojourns into the house to refill my glass of iced tea. The sun was far out over the ocean and just in the first stages of disappearing below the horizon. A gentle breeze from the west was stirring the leaves just enough to make a rustling sound as it wove a passage through the branches of the trees. It was a perfect day to barbecue and I planned to do just that. Marna had marinated the chicken and then I undertook the task of cooking the meat. Marna and the boys supervised my cooking. Instructions were given such as, "It's time to turn the chicken," "Be sure you cook it well," "Don't let it burn," and "Flames will scorch the meat." I proceeded to cook it the way they had always approved of in the past.

After eating, I was almost too uncomfortable to move but I was cajoled into playing catch with the boys. It was more or less a game of chase. I was having fun with my sons, and being together was the most important thing to me. After awhile, I decided it would make more sense to just watch the boys play and kibitz when the opportunity arose. I pulled up a lawn chair and sought comfort in just relaxing, observing, and commenting.

Marna was cleaning up the dishes as she monitored our activities from the kitchen window. Ever so thoughtful, Marna brought me a fresh glass of iced tea. I pulled up another lounge chair so she could join me. We enjoyed watching the boys and knew that they would sleep well this evening. About dusk, the phone rang. It was not for me but for Marna. I smiled and enjoyed the late afternoon even more.

It was early evening when the phone rang again. The odds were that it would be for me this time and it was. The answering service had a Dr. St. John on the phone and he was irritated. I asked the lady why he was disturbed and she said that he had a problem with his goat and needed to talk to or see a large animal veterinarian. He had called several that took cases on the peninsula but none could be located. It was not my intent to practice large animal medicine anymore as I was well entrenched in small animal practice. The service asked me if I would at least be available to consult him over the phone. I said, "Yes," and was immediately connected.

Dr. St. John was involved in a medical research project and was raising goats for the blood serum they produced to use in his studies. It was a genetic program. Therefore, it was necessary to raise goats and more importantly to perpetuate the bloodline to see if the immunity in his research could be passed transplacentally to the next generation. He wanted to talk to a veterinarian about the nanny that was kidding. He admitted that he did not have the skill to know how to assist her in a difficult birth.

I asked, "At what stage of delivery are we now?"

"Well, Doctor, there are two front legs showing."

"Is she straining?"

"Yes, she is pushing and I have been tugging on the two exposed feet."

"It doesn't sound very good."

"No, Doctor, it doesn't. Would you mind taking a look at her?"

"I will be there in about thirty minutes. Please have a bucket of hot water ready for me. I will have to stop at the hospital and pick up some instruments and medicine."

I took a long drink from my iced tea, got a sweaty hug from each of the boys, and a kiss from Marna. With all of the immediate responsibilities accomplished at home, I climbed into my Mustang and headed to the hospital on my way to the peninsula hills.

A map was carefully surveyed and I followed the instructions explicitly. Before long the number on the mailbox appeared. I pulled into the St. Johns' and parked my car near the barn. Dr. St. John came out of the house with a pail of hot water. Near the barn the nanny was tied to the fence with two legs protruding from her backside.

I carefully scrubbed up with surgical soap and then rinsed off well with the hot water. More of the soap was used to provide lubrication. The two legs that were protruding needed to be repelled. When this was accomplished, the nanny could be checked more thoroughly. The owner was correct. There were two front legs visible, but not from the same kid.

One foreleg was identified and the other front foot was located by tracing the first leg up to the chest and down the opposite leg. Both front legs were separated from all of the other feet. The kid's head, or rather the nose, was aligned with the forelegs. I grasped the two front feet in one hand and gave a tug of encouragement. A generous push by the nanny assisted me and a kid was born.

This procedure was repeated and the second kid arrived in the world. Dr. St. John was delighted—this goat had never had twins before. I smiled and told him he was in for a big surprise. In the same manner, the last of the triplets was exposed to the sunlight. Dr. St. John was overwhelmed! Number three was a cinch to deliver as it was not necessary to sort legs to locate the two front ones. An injection was given to the nanny to expel any retained afterbirth. As she was torn slightly during delivery I got an antibiotic and was filling the syringe. Dr. St. John requested that I not give that injection since there was a chance it would interfere with his experiments.

I washed and removed my OB gloves and then dumped my sundry supplies into the trunk of the car. Dr. St. John had disappeared into the house to write me a check. Both of the St. Johns returned from the house. His wife invited me to come in and have a cup of coffee and some cookies before I headed for home. We chatted for awhile and even took time to compare some of the unusual experiences that occurred in both human and animal medicine. Before I left the premises, I checked with the operator and found that there were no calls waiting.

The Mustang's engine turned over and I was just about ready to pull out of the driveway when Mrs. St. John hailed me to come into the house. I turned off the engine and walked up the back steps. I assumed that the answering service had called since I had left them that number so I could be reached. She had a package for me—some cookies for the boys. I thanked her and headed home.

I returned the supplies I had borrowed to the hospital. It had just turned dark and the lights of the house were on as I pulled into the driveway. I could see Marna's silhouette in the kitchen window. The boys were making a racket in the family room. I handed Marna the package of cookies for the boys. They would be dessert for the three boys after the evening meal. Three cookies of rather large proportions were handed out at mealtime. George requested the largest cookie so he was allowed to make his choice last. I didn't recall mentioning that I had three children to the St. Johns, but possibly I did and this would account for the three cookies. Again I may have been rewarded for the three kids that I had delivered.

After dinner I started to tell Marna about my day's experience, but before I could elaborate about it she suggested that I also share my story with the boys. They listened intently as I embellished the story with minute details and gesticulations. There was more than one question that followed and it was necessary to repeat parts of the story to provide the desired emphasis.

On "labor day" I had prearranged a visit back to the St. Johns for a recheck. This was to be a surprise visit for the boys. We arrived and were restricted from going into the barn—it was designated an aseptic area for his research program. Momma was led outside and her three kids followed her. The boys were delighted to see the kids but were not allowed to get close enough to pet them. The kids had something else on their agenda, for their momma represented dinner. All three headed for the nursing bag. One was left out—sort of like musical chairs. It was necessary to explain to the boys that the nanny could only feed two kids at a time because she had only two faucets. After the goat inspection, all five of us were invited into the kitchen to join them for cookies and milk.

All the boys could talk about on the way home was the goat farm. George and Albert even shared their experience at school during show-and-tell time. That goat farm visit was the dinner table topic for more than two weeks.

–10–

END OF THE TAIL

Often calls were just inquiries as to what to do. Owners needed to know whether immediate action was necessary or if their problem could be resolved the following day. At times it was difficult to relay my recommendations to the client. What seemed to be an emergency in their eyes was often not an emergency from a medical point of view. This scenario was posed to me one evening from clients who had noticed that worms were in their dog's stool. My conversation that evening was about a dog that the owners thought should have immediate attention for a very repulsive problem.

The lady initiated the call to me but immediately turned the receiver over to her husband once she knew that she was talking to a veterinarian.

"May I help you?" I inquired.

"Doctor, my dog has worms."

I asked if the worms were seen on their dog or were they noticed on their dog's stool.

"My wife noticed them on Frieda's poop in the backyard and almost got sick to her stomach."

"How long had the stool been in the backyard?"

"Honey, how long would you say the stool had been in the backyard?" was the question I heard over the phone.

"She cleaned up the poop about three days ago so I would guess about seventy-two hours."

"Did she notice if the worms had little black spots on their head ends?"

"Doc, you've got to be kidding. Once she saw the worms she wouldn't even go out into the backyard to empty the garbage. My wife would prob-ably barf if I even suggested that she look at them that closely. Why all the questions? I just want to bring Frieda in for worming now!"

I said, "I am quizzing you because I am trying to determine if what you see on the stool are worms or maggots. Maggots have little black spots on their heads and tapeworms do not. Maggots are the larvae of flies and are unrelated to worms. Maggots may be found on the stool as early as twenty-four hours if the stool is not picked up and the weather conditions are favorable."

It was necessary to explain that whether worms or maggots were seen, the problem did not need to be addressed that evening. I recommended that he pick up a stool sample from the yard, put it into a plastic bag and drop it off at his veterinarian's office in the morning. The office would do some laboratory work and advise them accordingly.

Marna was in the kitchen listening to this conversation and the boys were exposed to it as well for they were setting the table. The family often overheard my conversations with clients. Allen said that he was glad that I was not at the dinner table talking over a portable phone. The rest of the family agreed with his comment. I was cognizant that some client conver-sations are not dinner subjects, and I tried to avoid these. On occasion, I did get carried away and went into considerable more detail about my happenings during office hours. I could always tell when too much was said—the boys would not interrupt me but they would look blankly at each other.

Just as we finished dessert, my first emergency call came in. The Raymonds had a Labrador that had a severe tail injury. Their dog needed immediate attention. The car door had been slammed on Chester's tail and it was bleeding profusely. I recommended that they apply pressure to the tail to slow down the bleeding, wrap the tail in a bandage or towel so Chester would not "wag" blood all over the car, and then head for the hospital.

When the Raymonds arrived at the hospital, their clothes were spotted with blood. En route, the blood from the additional tail wagging was added to the blood spots they had received earlier as they were attempting to bandage the tail. Chester had persisted in wagging his tail, and, needless to say, blood was everywhere. Most dogs love to wag their tails and Chester was no exception. It was impossible to hold the tail still, so Chester was sedated with surital. Mrs. Raymond borrowed some towels to clean up both the car and herself while her husband assisted me. I gave her a bottle of hydrogen peroxide to clean up any bloodstains on her clothing that would not respond to water treatment.

The last two inches of the tail had almost been severed. Mr. Raymond was now able to leave me and assist his wife in cleaning the inside of their car. I trimmed the hair from the tip of the tail, scrubbed the surgical area down, and prepared for surgery. I removed the portion of the tail that had lost its vascularity, ligated the necessary vessels, and sutured him up.

They completed the car-cleaning job and I finished surgery at about the same time. I ushered the Raymonds into the washroom and they started the job of cleaning themselves up. I bandaged the tail with ample elastic tape. My patient was dismissed. He was not to be bathed for three days. An appointment for a recheck was made. The loss of the end of his tail would never impede his wag but he would be a slightly shorter dog from head to tail.

—11—

NEIGHBORHOOD
TOMCAT

J ust before dawn I was behind the wheel of my Mustang. My patient had a wound on her thigh. It had been described as a possible gunshot wound. They informed me in detail about how all of the youngsters in the neighborhood owned pellet guns and had the propensity to shoot at anything that moved. I listened patiently at their speculation while making up the medical record. Rooter, a Labrador, did not seem to be annoyed by the lesion. He was more interested in watching me and that was rather unusual for any pet that came in on an emergency.

Together we put Rooter up on the exam table, and the owners then restrained her while I inspected the wound. The area around the lesion was moist from the serum that was oozing from it. Rooter was so active and unmanageable that there was no way I could examine her without sedation. This was given. When Rooter was relaxed sufficiently that she was lying on her side, I was able to begin my examination.

The wound was probed. No passageway could be located that would indicate she had been hit by a bullet or pellet. The owners reaffirmed their suspicions that Rooter had indeed been shot by some mischievous youngster. I did not wish to argue; it would only make matters worse in my relationship with them if they were right and I was wrong. The only way to confirm if there was a foreign body present in Rooter's thigh was to take an x-ray. We loaded her on a cart and rolled her into the x-ray room. Two views were taken and no foreign body was evident. All of us were relieved.

Even though Rooter was not fully awake and rather sluggish, we decided that it would be prudent to send her home. It took two of us to lift her off the cart and then to put her into the van.

On the way out to the van, curiosity got the better of me and I just had to inquire as to how the name of Rooter was selected for their Lab. They had owned her mother, and when Rooter was only two weeks old, she had climbed into a backyard area drain and became lodged in it. They tried to get her out and couldn't without the possibility of injuring her so they called the Roto-Rooter man to assist with the problem. He had to dig up almost six feet of lawn and break out some drain tile before he could get her out safely. They were so appreciative of his efforts that they promised to name her after him. They didn't quite do that but they did name her "Rooter."

When I arrived home, Marna informed me that the operator had called and wanted me to call back. A client was having some problem with a prescription. I called the answering service and was given the telephone number of the client. Her dog had chewed up her prescription vial with some medication in it. She could not identify the medication. The only thing she could read on the chewed up vial was "keep out of reach of children." I called the pharmacy to learn more about the medication. They were able to trace the prescription and give me the name and the number of tablets dispensed. I called the lady back and asked her how many had already been taken and how many had been recovered from the floor. It was now easy to determine how many tablets were not accounted for. I called the Poison Control Center for their assistance.

The Poison Control Center recommended an emetic followed in half an hour with a gastric antacid that would give soothing relief to the stomach. I asked the owner to bring her dog to the hospital so that I could carry out the recommendation of the poison center. We met at the hospital and I followed the instructions. I used a narcotic tablet called apomorphine as my emetic of choice. A tablet of this product is placed in the conjunctival area of the eye. The response was immediate and effective. To stop the vomiting I irrigated the eye with a saline solution and whatever remained of the tablet was washed away. Mission accomplished! We waited the prescribed half-hour to insure that all of the apomorphine in the bloodstream was utilized before we squirted mylanta into his mouth to neutralize the stomach.

Later that evening the lady called back and wondered when she could feed her dog and what type of food she should offer it. I recommended cottage cheese and boiled rice for two consecutive meals and then his regular diet if no further symptoms developed.

I was on the road once more this evening. Mr. Vargus called me about his cat, Tonto, who had an injured left eye. Mr. Vargus described the problem in detail and I realized immediately that it was not a simple problem. They lived about a block away from us and owned a cat that was a neighborhood problem. I recognized Tonto immediately when he was placed on the exam table. He was a huge black and white male cat with a scarred head and torn ears. He had no neck at all so it was impossible to even grab him by the nape of the neck. He had big yellow eyes that would glare at you and suggest that he would be willing to fight anyone anytime. Tonight he was glaring at me with only one eye because his left eye was closed and draining a bloody fluid.

Tonto had a reputation that extended for several blocks. He would roam the area at night, howl at the moon, and fight any other tomcat that would look at him. Since tomcats establish regions or domains and all queens in that area are part of their harem, any tomcat that entered Tonto's area needed to be driven off. Tonto was so dominant that I was certain he was always encroaching on other male cats' areas in order to enlarge his own harem.

Marna told me several times about the big black and white cat that would come up to our back porch screen and mark his territory. No matter how well she cleaned the screen some of the stench lingered. Any cat that entered Tonto's territory was an immediate challenge to him. These fights for dominance could be heard for some distance but they always seemed as if they were just below our bedroom window. Tonto's nocturnal habits were not appreciated.

Tonto was placed on the exam table and I made a valiant effort to examine his injured eye. He would not cooperate. We had a confrontation. I wanted to be in charge and he already assumed that he was in charge. He was challenging me—his ears were laid back along his head and he gave a deep growl. Every time my hand was extended his claws were extended. It was a standoff and he appeared to be in control. We even tried to wrap him in a blanket so I could examine him without getting my hands scratched or bitten. Each time we tried to wrap a blanket around him, he would bat it away and snarl. It was now necessary for all of us to be extra cautious—Tonto was seething mad.

After several attempts, we were eventually able to cover him with a blanket and then administer a sedative mixture of ketamine and acepromazine through the blanket into a muscle on his rear leg. Ten minutes later he was a nice kitty cat. I could pet him without inciting him. I was now in control! It was time for me to evaluate the damaged eye. I held the eye lid open with a retractor and found that the structure of the left eye was completely destroyed. The eye was damaged so badly that what remained of the eye needed to be removed. Tonto would have vision from only his right eye in the future.

Since Tonto was already under sedation and very difficult to manage when he was awake, we felt it would be prudent to take him into surgery right away rather than wait until morning. The surgical area was prepared and draped. Before I gloved up, Mr. Vargus decided he would go home, so I locked him out of the hospital. He would wait for my follow-up call at home when the surgery was completed.

I enucleated the eye, and when the mass was removed and put on the surgical tray, there was a definite "plunk" sound. This noise puzzled me, for soft tissue isn't likely to make any sound at all. When surgery was completed and Tonto was situated in his recovery cage, I returned to surgery to investigate the tissue mass that had been removed. Carefully I examined the mass and exposed a lead ball. At first it appeared to be a ball bearing but on closer evaluation, I realized it was a cast lead ball like one used in a muzzle-loaded gun.

The Vargus family was called and I gave them the postsurgery report and described the size of the lead ball. I suggested to Mr. Vargus that it would be a good time to castrate Tonto as he was still under the effect of the anesthetic and he would be easy to handle. Mr. Vargus was vehemently opposed to this type of surgery.

While I was cleaning up the surgery, Mr. Vargus knocked on the door to attract my attention. He wanted to see the lead ball that had caused all of the damage. At first we rationalized that Tonto had been shot. Then we realized that if it had come from a gun, the ball would have penetrated much more deeply and Tonto would not have survived. It could not have been thrown hard enough to penetrate that deeply, so after all of these possibilities we agreed on a slingshot as the weapon for two reasons. The velocity of the ball would account for that degree of damage and Mr. Vargus had never heard any gunshot sounds in the neighborhood. We also felt that some youth was more likely to own a slingshot. If our analysis was correct, it was a very accurate and lucky shot.

The hospital discharged Tonto in a few days. His habits continued as before. He acted like he had only taken a vacation, for he continued to roam the neighborhood. Marna routinely hosed off the screen. Sounds of cat fights in the wee hours of the morning were still prevalent and annoyed those who were within earshot of the squabble. The local residents spoke of seeing a big black and white cat everywhere. I hoped that the residents were seeing some of Tonto's descendants, for he was dominant enough to have sired many offspring.

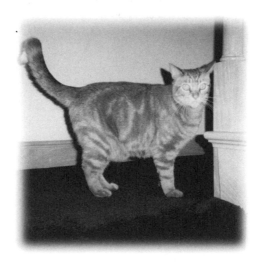

–12–

HAND IN MOUTH

The next dog that visited me for emergency care was a vizsla named Mac. Mac was a fairly large dog so I offered to help lift him up on the exam table. Mr. Jacobs said, "No, I'd better lift him!" Caution signs went up—I realized that he probably was not too friendly a dog.

Mac's digestive system was out of whack. He had been expelling gas intermittently with diarrhea. This had been going on for a little over a week. The problem had gotten better and then worse—then better again. Now it was worse. The diarrhea problem needed to be corrected. The family did not know when to bring him into their house or to leave him outside. Most of the time, it seemed, he was in the house when he should have been out.

I inserted a thermometer in the appropriate place and that immediately stimulated a bowel movement. A fecal sample was collected, the table cleaned up, and the examination was started all over again. I turned on the exhaust fan for obvious reasons. Mac's temperature was normal. He was straining intermittently and I reminded myself not to stand directly behind him.

Next I planned to listen to his chest and abdomen. Just as I placed the stethoscope on his chest, he turned his head and grabbed my hand in his mouth. He didn't really bite me but held my hand in his mouth firmly enough that he let me know I had better leave it there rather than ripping it out of his mouth. Mr. Jacobs laughed and said that that was a game Mac played. "He won't let go until I ask him to let go," Mr. Jacobs explained. I then asked Mr. Jacobs if he would be so kind as to ask Mac to release my hand. He commanded, "Let go, Mac." My hand was free. I gave my hand a cursory check and the skin wasn't even broken. The only thing I had to do was to wash the saliva off and dry my hand. Mr. Jacobs said that Mac sometimes did that to him when he was petting him. I wondered what would be the outcome if Mac grabbed someone's hand and that person did not know the release command.

I gave Mac a GI cocktail very carefully to avoid a repeat experience. I suggested that Mac be taken outside and walked around since I did not want to clean up any problems. I really wanted to get the dog out of the hospital as soon as possible. While Mac was being walked, I had the opportunity to check the fecal sample under the microscope. Several ova from whipworms were evident. I gave Mr. Jacobs instructions for overnight care and made an appointment for Mac in the morning when the office first opened in the morning.

When Mr. Jacobs and Mac were gone, I carefully reexamined my hand and still could not believe that there wasn't even a tooth impression on it. What a soft mouth the vizsla had. I was happy about the results.

My next case directed me to the Lawndale hospital. A little mixed-breed puppy was brought in with a very sore neck. From the moment it came into the hospital, it was scratching its neck. The rear leg looked as if was in perpetual motion and the neck was raw and oozing. The owners were perplexed and expressed their fears to me that the pup might have some dreadful skin disease. They were afraid to even pet the pup for fear that whatever it had might be transmitted to humans. I filled out the facts on the medical record and recorded "No Name" where ordinarily the animal's given name was entered. The owners were planning to sell or give the pup away but could not find anyone interested in a pup with a sore neck. No one wanted to buy problems.

I examined the rash more astutely—it was unusual because it extended completely around the neck. The lesion was wet and very sore everywhere the rear feet could reach. Not only was the rash very evident, but the entire neck area was extremely swollen, giving the appearance of no neck at all. Somewhere in my memory bank I remembered reading about a similar case. I asked the owners if they had ever put a collar on the puppy. They said, "Yes." "What happened to the collar?" I asked. Neither of the owners had a satisfactory answer. "She may have lost it," came the latent reply. I related to the owners that the collar might still be on the neck. Possibly as the pup increased in size, the skin grew completely over the collar and now the collar was hidden from view. This was a very difficult scenario for them to believe.

I recommended that it would be best to make a nick in the skin to see if my guess was correct. The owners agreed to this procedure. Lo and behold, I felt the scalpel hit something hard. Investigating further, I was able to expose what did appear to be a plastic flea collar. Finally, I was able to confirm that the collar was definitely the culprit. The swelling was due to the fact that the collar was too snug on the neck and the chemicals contained within the collar had caused an adverse reaction.

No Name was given several whiffs of an inhalant anesthetic and I went to work. I clipped, scrubbed, and painted the neck with antiseptic. The neck was then palpated carefully to locate the buckle. An incision was made over the buckle and extended until the buckle was entirely exposed. The collar was then cut in two. I grasped the buckle with forceps, and with a little gentle tugging the buckle end of the collar slid out. With the buckle held firmly in the forceps' grip, I carried the trophy to the front of the hospital to show it off to the owners. They looked in disbelief.

The anesthetic was wearing off so I hurriedly rubbed some forte salve, which contained cortisone, into the neck area and gave injections of both amoxicillin and azium to alleviate any possibility of infection and to reduce the swelling. No Name was then put into a cage with the thought in mind that he would be discharged the next day if the neck was showing the anticipated signs of improvement.

As the owners exited the hospital, they were shaking their heads about the event that had taken place that evening. I was shaking my head also. Some people really do not pay any attention to their pet's welfare. The owners probably expected the collar to stretch as the pup matured. More than likely, the flea collar was put on No Name and they just forgot about it. I hoped that the neck would heal properly. It was now likely that new owners could be found and that they would provide better care and give the pup a more plausible name.

−13−

GRAND CENTRAL
STATION

This Sunday was very different from past Sundays. It was summer and several of my colleagues were on vacation. I had made arrangements to take care of their cases while they were away. That day I was to do morning treatments. I had three hospitals to visit, which meant some traveling.

Late to bed and early to rise was my plan. Marna was already up too and had coffee waiting for me when I arrived in the kitchen. The boys slowly began to appear in the kitchen. Albert wanted cinnamon waffles this morning. Greta greeted me as I walked out the back door and headed for the Mustang. In the background the boys began chanting, "Waffles, waffles, waffles." I could almost smell the cinnamon as I pulled out of the driveway and headed for Hawthorne.

Morning treatments were done at Hawthorne, San Pedro, and Redondo Beach. It was much easier to get up and do treatments early because the kennel staffs were usually present and that enabled me to have some assistance in managing the pets while I performed the necessary tasks. Before I had completed my last case, the answering service located me. A car accident case at the San Pedro hospital needed care. I left moments later and the kennel staff obliged me by cleaning up the mess that I had left. It is infrequent that cases occur at the hospital where I am heading, and I was thankful that this was the situation that morning.

It was a long drive to the harbor and the clients were there only a minute or two ahead of me. We rushed the Scottie into the treatment

room. I set up an IV drip and added solu-delta-cortef injection of a
steroid to the solution to counteract shock. Bozo had been hit by a car.
The car had then passed over him to the horror of the owners who were
standing nearby. Bozo had definitely been tumbled under the car, and
the owners were not certain whether the tires had actually run over
him or not.

My examination continued. Two teeth were missing and he was
bleeding from his mouth. I cleared the clotted blood from his mouth to
establish a better passage of air. Carefully, I examined his body, being
cautious in case further injuries were present. I gently lifted the left rear
leg, and Bozo objected by raising his head slightly and whimpering. I
became even more cautious as I lifted the leg slightly and then rotated it.
A more profound response was elicited from Bozo. With this information,
I explained to the Collinses that there appeared to be a fracture of the
femur and very likely a pelvic fracture as well. Permission was authorized
to proceed with the necessary x-rays.

At this stage, it was impossible to take the proper views of the leg and
pelvis because Bozo was alert enough to feel pain and it was not good
judgment to sedate him because he was still showing signs of shock. Ever
so slowly his pulse improved and his color returned to the mucous
membranes in his mouth. We monitored him for awhile and he gradually
overcame the initial shock stage. He slowly raised his head in response to
his owners' voices. It was best for Bozo to be still, for any movement might
cause further damage. Finally it was possible to administer a mild sedative
intravenously until he was resting comfortably. The radiographs
confirmed fractures of the femur and the ilium of the pelvis. The leg was
splinted and Bozo was hospitalized with the intravenous solution of saline
and dextrose to support him still connected.

After Bozo was comfortably located in his cage, we returned to the
reception room and the pertinent information about Bozo was recorded in
his medical record. I chatted with the Collinses for a bit in the back room,
but being curious, I still had a lot of questions. Finally I got around to the
question, "How did this accident happen?" The Collinses had been
playing ball with Bozo in the front yard—a game of throw and fetch. A
long throw had been made and Bozo chased the ball out into the street
where he was hit by a car. "You know what made us mad? The driver
didn't even stop!"

We checked on Bozo once more and noted that he was resting well. I would be checking on him periodically the rest of the day. More x-rays would be taken by the resident veterinarian in the morning and corrective surgery would follow. I asked the Collinses to call in the morning for a progress report and a surgery schedule. In the meantime, I assured the Collinses that I would call and let them know how their dog was doing when I did my follow-up.

While Bozo was being treated, Marna had reached me by phone. There was a case in Manhattan Beach that needed attention. I asked the service to call the client and tell them that I would be at that hospital in about twenty minutes. I left immediately even though the hospital was only partially cleaned up; I would clean up later when I returned to check on Bozo.

Marna was indispensable, for she was my personal answering service for the commercial answering services. She always knew where I was and where I was headed because I kept in close contact with her by phone. If one of the four services called home for me, Marna would phone me and then I would call that operator back. Allen was her substitute and he did a remarkable job in keeping track of me also.

As I pulled into the parking lot at the Manhattan hospital, a car pulled in behind me. A lady jumped out of her car and came running over to me before I could turn off the ignition. Her husband was getting their whippet from the backseat. She said, "I think my dog is already dead. He was hit by a car about ten minutes ago and hasn't moved since." I ushered them immediately into the exam room. I placed a stethoscope over the dog's chest and heard absolutely nothing. The tongue was blue, the eyes were glazed, and no pulse could be found. I informed them that their dog was indeed dead.

Before I knew it, someone was coming in the front door with a cat. The emergency room looked like Grand Central Station. The owners of the feline informed me that the answering service had told them to come to this hospital. I escorted them into the second exam room and then returned to the party who had just lost their dog.

The owners of the expired dog wished to know what to do with their pet. I informed them that I could take care of the arrangements if that was their desire. "You are not going to experiment with him, are you?" the lady asked. "Absolutely not!" I responded. "We have an agency that will pick him up." "Then what happens to him?" the man asked. "The agency will cremate him." The owners seemed satisfied. They took care of their account, thanked me, and left in tears.

The operator called me to tell me that another case was on the way. A dog had been hit by a car and was in bad shape. They had directed them to this hospital because they knew I would soon be there. I thanked them for their foresight and told them that the accident case had already arrived and that the owners were just leaving. The second case with the feline that was scheduled had arrived after the surprise accident case. The reception room was becoming an even busier Grand Central Station.

It was now necessary to pay attention to the clients who were waiting in the second exam room with their cat. Information was provided by the Farrels about their tomcat, Mischief. Mischief looked out of balance with his lopsided face where large swelling was evident. He had been in a fight a couple of days ago and this abscess was the result of that skirmish.

The abscess needed to be lanced—a rather messy operation, and abscesses have a tendency to drain considerably so I recommended that Mischief stay overnight. I instructed the Farrels to call in the morning to check on their cat and find out what time he would be released. Mischief would be given a clean-up bath prior to discharge so it would be likely that the Farrels could pick him up on their way home from work. When I treat abscesses in a full male cat, I usually suggest that owners have their cat altered sometime in the future in order to avoid a repeat problem.

The Farrels left and I went to work. Mischief was sedated with surital. The abscess was lanced and then drained. It was then flushed with a weak solution of iodine, and a seton (a drain in a lesion tied back on itself) was placed to keep the incision open so it would continue to drain. An injection of penicillin followed and Mischief was put into his hotel cage for the night.

It was midafternoon now, and I was very hungry. I stopped at the local fast-food restaurant for a hamburger and a soft drink, and then headed for home. The boys were playing in the backyard so I pulled up a lounge chair and settled into it with my belated lunch. The boys had located a couple of pieces of pipe and some horseshoes. The pipes were driven into the ground about twenty feet apart and they were having quite a session making up the rules to play a game. Allen was obviously in charge—his decisions appeared to be final.

A few minutes later Marna joined me. We sat there and watched our three sons. On occasion some of their disputes needed to be arbitrated. Marna returned to the kitchen and soon reappeared with snacks and beverages for all of us. I relaxed on the lounge chair anticipating my next emergency. Waiting for a call was not necessarily a good idea, for an emergency never seemed to happen when expected. They always seemed to occur when least desired or anticipated. I made several visits to check on Bozo during the evening and night. I checked on him again in the morning before I went to my daytime relief commitment. Bozo looked rather uncomfortable but appeared to be resting well. I connected another liter of fluid and left for my daily routine.

14

THE CAR
ALWAYS WINS

Car accident cases were more numerous than normal that week, and I was on my way again to Hawthorne for another car accident emergency. The owners had informed me over the phone that their cat had an apparent head injury. They had heard tires screech about an hour ago and later Sweetie was found on the front porch. Their cat was unable to walk now and seemed disoriented.

We all arrived at the hospital at the same time. Sweetie appeared to be oblivious to all that was happening around her. I immediately noted several problems. Her jaw was malaligned. After careful scrutiny, I determined that she also had a split or rent in her hard palate in the top of her mouth. This type of injury was common place for a cat competing with a car. The car would always win.

Since it was a three-day weekend, I explained to the owners that I would not do surgery right away in case there was a mild concussion. I would do the corrective surgery tomorrow or the next day depending on her progress. I told the owners that while Sweetie remained in the hospital, I would call them daily and give them a progress report. On the second day Sweetie had improved enough for me to proceed with corrective surgery. I called the Winslows and told them of my decision. They wanted to come right down and wait at the hospital while I was in surgery. There was no advantage for the owners to stay there while surgery was being performed and I promised to call them when Sweetie was put back together again.

A short-acting anesthetic was given and an endotrachial tube was passed in order to put her on the gas machine. Instruments and supplies that were needed for that night's surgery were placed on the mayo surgical tray. I was now prepared for surgery.

Closing the tear in the hard palate was first. It was difficult to adequately get to as the endotrachial tube from the gas machine was in the way. A speculum was also used to keep the mouth open wide and it too competed for space in the cat's small mouth. When this part of the surgery was completed, I turned to the next repair job. The jaw was not technically fractured; it was separated at the mandibular symphysis where the two halves of the body are fused together forming a weaker place in the bone structure of the jaw. I realigned the jaw. Then the jaw was securely wired by wrapping the wire behind the canine teeth so the wire would not slip off. The jaw would remain wired in that position for three to four weeks until the mandible "fused" again.

Sweetie was put into a cage and the intravenous feeding was slowed down to one drop every six seconds. I cleaned the instruments and then put them back into the sterile solution. The surgery and treatment rooms sparkled when I finished cleaning them. I called Marna so she would know where I would be and then I called the owners and gave them an update on Sweetie.

Sweetie would be a lot better in a couple of days when the pain and swelling diminished. I predicted that she would be able to be discharged as soon as she was capable of eating on her own. Her care would be in the hands of the doctor who came in the morning, so I asked the Winslows to call in the morning when the hospital opened.

Before I left to go home the phone rang and Marna was on the other end of the line. Faux Pas, our own cat, had just been hit by a car. Marna asked me to wait at the hospital and she would be there as soon as possible. About all I could do was to unlock the front door and wait. I thought that waiting is what clients had to do when they had an injured pet. Waiting was not easy. I couldn't even predict her injuries, for Marna gave me no clues.

Marna burst in the front door with Faux Pas in her arms and took her directly into the treatment room. Our cat was gasping for breath. I inserted an endotracheal tube and hooked Faux Pas to the oxygen machine. I squeezed the bag to correspond to her normal respiratory rhythm. Her color improved and her breathing became deeper and more regular than before. Marna stood in the doorway and was crying. I solicited my crying wife to pump the oxygen bag as I had done so my hands would be free to examine Faux Pas more efficiently. No fractures were noted. Her breathing was still a problem.

I listened carefully to her chest and heard intestinal sounds. The next step was to take an x-ray of her thorax. My suspicions were confirmed— Faux Pas had a diaphragmatic hernia. Her diaphragm had ruptured on impact with the car and her intestines were now positioned around the heart and lungs. This interference with normal lung expansion had caused the respiratory problem. Surgery had to be done now, for if we took her off positive respiration she would surely die.

All this time Marna had been helping Faux Pas breathe by squeezing the oxygen bag. I informed Marna of the impending surgery and that it would be necessary for her to continue helping our cat breathe during surgery. I needed her assistance during surgery because the thoracic cavity was to be exposed and Faux Pas's normal breathing would have to compete with the outside air pressure. Marna gave me sort of a wistful look, but she knew she had to help—there was no one else present. Her job was to rhythmically pump the oxygen bag on the anesthetic machine. She was to count out loud—one, two, three, four—squeeze the bag firmly but slowly and then allow the bag to refill, and then keep repeating the procedure until surgery was completed. Marna could not watch. She sat on a stool and faced the opposite direction throughout the surgical proce-dure.

One, two, three, four—surgery was started. This only sound in the room was continually repeated. It almost drove me crazy but it was neces-sary to maintain the rhythm. Faux Pas's chest and abdominal cavities were exposed and I placed the intestines back into his abdominal cavity. One, two, three, four—Marna was doing a great job.

The diaphragm was repaired first. I then closed the chest and abdom-inal cavities with sutures. Marna wanted to know if her job was done. "Not yet," was my response. Negative pressure still had to be reestablished in the chest. Using a syringe with a large needle, I carefully penetrated the thorax while avoiding the heart and lungs. About twenty milliliters of air was aspirated. Negative pressure had now been established. Faux Pas was now breathing on her own.

Marna's job was completed. The room was quiet. The oxygen supply on the anesthetic machine was turned off. I didn't have a chance to take off my surgical gloves when Marna broke into tears. I got a great hug from her and I hugged her back. We then put our cat into a critical care observation cage so we could keep an eye on her for awhile.

While I was cleaning up, Marna put on some coffee. When it was through brewing, we sat down, took a deep breath, and just relaxed. We had taken only a few sips of coffee when Marna remembered to call home and tell our boys that Faux Pas would be okay.

My question was, "What happened?" Faux Pas had a habit of crossing the street to the neighbor's house in order to watch the goldfish in their pond. Sometimes she would sit there for hours just watching with only her head moving as the fish swam by. Our cat was either venturing over or returning from the pond when she was hit. Marna saw a car stop abruptly and people get out. When she went outside to investigate, she heard the driver say, "I think I just hit someone's cat." Marna looked around and saw Faux Pas lying in the ivy alongside the street. Marna picked up Faux Pas. She asked a neighbor to watch the boys and called me before heading to the hospital.

We finished our coffee, poured another cup, and then set about cleaning up the hospital as a team. It was nice to have someone help me with this chore. It required a little longer time to clean up that night as we took numerous coffee breaks. When we finally got home, we reassured the boys that Faux Pas would be home in a day or two.

—15—

ONE FIGHT— TWO PATIENTS

Two telephone calls came in from the answering service minutes apart. Both emergencies came from the same hospital's exchange. The first party had a German shepherd with a lacerated face. I informed them that I would be at the hospital in Lawndale in approximately fifteen minutes. The second party was scheduled to be there forty-five minutes after the first case.

When I arrived at Lawndale, a German shepherd was being walked around on its leash by the owners.

After obtaining the pertinent data we proceeded into the exam room. The shepherd had numerous puncture wounds on its muzzle and some other minor wounds around its neck. The cheek and part of the lip were badly swollen and very tender to touch. The owner held the dog in such a manner that he could not bite me. (When examining any pet's facial area, it is necessary to be cautious.) The dog objected to my examination considerably but the owner did a great job in restraining the pet. No stitches were required. My main concern was the possibility of infection, so the antibiotic, lincomycin, was administered and a prescription of the same product was sent home. The owner then lifted the dog off the table, and as soon as he had all four feet on the floor he turned and growled at me showing his teeth.

The owners explained that they had been walking their dog on the beach when this pit bull came out of nowhere. "A rough and tumble fight occurred and the end result was that his pit bull grabbed my dog by the nose or face and was shaking him. The other owner arrived on the scene and the two of us were able to separate the dogs without being bitten ourselves. I grabbed my dog's leash and the other party retrieved the leash on his dog. A few unpleasant remarks were made and we departed. I don't know why people let their dogs run loose," was the shepherd owner's final comment.

I stepped out of the exam room and closed the door. As the prescription was being filled my other emergency arrived and they were escorted to exam room number two. "As soon as I am through with the client in the other exam room, I'll be with you," I said as I closed their door. When the prescription was filled, I returned to the shepherd's owner and explained how the medication was to be given. The business part of the evening was then completed and the party left.

In the second exam room a pit bull was already on the exam table waiting for my attention. There was a deep laceration on its shoulder that required suturing. I explained to the owners that if they could restrain their dog properly so that I didn't have to be concerned with him grabbing me, I could block the wound locally and then suture it without having to give a general anesthetic. They confirmed that they could manage their dog and I went to work. A local block of xylocaine was given to numb the damaged shoulder. The hair was clipped and the skin debrided. When the dog indicated to me that he felt no pain, I knew that I could safely suture the lesion. I gave the pit bull a friendly pat as I completed the last of five stitches and the owner lifted the dog from the table and gently placed him on the floor.

The owner continued our intermittent conversation by saying, "I don't know why owners allow their pets to run loose on the beach." I began to put two and two together but made no comments. The owner continued the conversation further by telling me that his dog was on a leash but had gotten loose and a big German shepherd had attacked him.

The account was settled and I returned to the exam rooms to clean up. I thought for some time about the two cases that I had just treated and tried to concoct a story of my own that would plausibly describe the circumstances that led up to the confrontation. Both dogs had leashes on them because that is how the owners separated them. The other dog had been running loose according to each of the owners. It was unlawful to have unleashed dogs running loose on the beach. Each owner probably released their grip on the leash in order to allow their dogs to have a little more freedom and get more exercise. If the beach patrol stopped them, they could claim that their dog broke free from their grip on the leash and that they were only trying to catch him. If my analysis was correct, each owner paid the penalty in veterinary services that day.

A trip to Redondo Beach was next on my evening's agenda. Mrs. Chan was already on her way with an injured cat. I drove over to Manhattan Beach on the way to check on a case from earlier in the day. This fall night had turned cooler once the sun had settled below the western horizon. Clouds were accumulating and beginning to billow in from over the ocean. The air smelled as if it were about to rain. By the time I had seen my interim patient and returned to my Mustang, a misty rain had commenced. It was the first rain of the year and the smell of dust being settled was a refreshing odor.

Mrs. Chan arrived at the hospital with her cat and we went immediately into the exam room. I began my examination by inserting a rectal thermometer. I picked up CoCo's tail to steady her so the thermometer could be recovered. A large patch of loose skin fell forward. This piece of skin was about four inches long and an inch wide. A comparable area of exposed flesh was now visible. I looked up to say something to Mrs. Chan. She wasn't there. She had disappeared. Apparently, she had leaned against the wall for support and then silently slid down the wall and was now comfortably resting on the floor in a sitting position. She had passed out and was motionless. I quickly put CoCo into a cage and returned to help my other "patient" on this rainy evening.

It required a few minutes for Mrs. Chan to return to the real world, and when she was able, I assisted her into the doctor's office where there was a day couch for her to lie down. I knew that even if she was able to walk in a half an hour, there was no way I would trust her to drive home. I called Marna to come to my aid and then attended to Mrs. Chan as best I could. Her feet were propped up, and I asked her to remain on the couch and not try to get up until my wife arrived to assist her.

While Mrs. Chan was resting comfortably in the office, kitty was removed from her cage and examined with more scrutiny. The loose flap of skin was not viable and would have to be removed. After I made this decision, I returned to the office to discuss the needed surgery with the kitty's owner. Permission to do the surgery was granted. At this point, Marna arrived and helped me by getting all of the necessary medical information from Mrs. Chan. Marna was sitting on a chair and Mrs. Chan was reclining on the couch. The scene reminded me of a psychologist talking to a patient. Marna volunteered to take Mrs. Chan home in our car. While Marna was being a chauffeur, I would get everything ready for the coming surgery.

Marna was back from her trip in no time at all. I entubated CoCo and introduced her to the gas anesthetic machine. Her fur was trimmed around the lesion and the skin was then painted with an antiseptic solution. Drapes were then used to provide a sterile field. I began surgery. The nonvital tissue was debrided and the opposing tissue was united as the wound was closed. Necessary retention stitches were used to take some of the tension from the suture line. Surgery was now completed.

Marna was a great help. She never liked to assist me in surgery for she claimed that I was not polite to her. Instead of asking her to "please hand me this" or to "please get me that," I was too concise. I would say "sponges," "suture material," "forceps," etc. She felt that I was ordering her around instead of kindly asking for her assistance. And so it was!

We cleaned up the premises and then Marna drove the Chan car to her house while I followed in the Mustang. We returned to the hospital and Marna retrieved her car. As she pulled out of the parking lot, she rolled down her window and said, "Meet you at the yogurt place down the street." Before I had a chance to respond she had taken off.

We placed our order and found a table. I remarked that the laceration on the Chan cat was one of the worse I had ever seen. Marna asked, "Do you know the story behind it?" I did not. Marna then related to me what had happened as told by Mrs. Chan when they were together in our car.

"Mrs. Chan had gotten into her car about a half-hour after returning from the grocery store. When she started the engine this time, she heard a funny sound followed by a frightened cry from a cat. The noise was muted and seemed to come from under her car's hood. She immediately got out of her car with the intention of raising the hood to investigate the sound she heard. As soon as the engine was turned off, her cat ran out from under the car and headed for the front porch. When Mrs. Chan got to the porch, CoCo was huddled by the back door bleeding. She went into the house, got a towel, and wrapped up her cat. Then she called the hospital. You know the rest," Marna said.

We finished our yogurt and realized that the boys were missing out on this snack so we purchased a quart to take home. Marna drove home in her car and I followed. Only Allen was still up so he had his dish. Marna used the excuse that it was not polite for him to sit and eat while we watched, so we enjoyed a small second helping and a cup of coffee in his presence. The rest was saved for George and Albert.

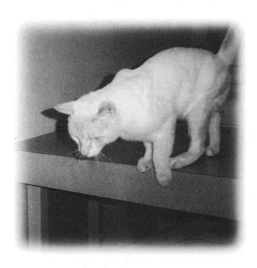

—16—

BOBTAILED CAT

It was a pleasant weekend afternoon and George, my middle son, and I were sitting in the backyard, soaking up sunshine. We were watching big white puffs of clouds sailing across the sky behind an ever so gentle sea breeze. Our chat was interrupted by a call from a gentleman who had an injured cat and wanted to meet me at the Manhattan Beach hospital. George wanted to go with me so I had him check with Marna. Permission was granted and we were on our way.

As we drove up the coast we could see several sailboats out in the ocean, and George immediately compared them to the clouds that we had been watching earlier. One cloud that he now saw was moving faster than another, and George wondered how long it would take for it to catch the one it appeared to be chasing. He likened it to a pirate trying to overhaul a treasure ship. George's imagination had just about played out as we pulled into the hospital parking lot.

Mr. Clark had a cat named Amigo with him that had an injured tail. The skin from about halfway down the tail to the very tip was completely gone. Very little hemorrhaging had occurred and that which had occurred was cleaned up by Amigo who was constantly licking it. I looked up at Mr. Clark. He must have sensed what I was about to ask because he offered, "My neighbor's dog got him by the tail but he was able to get away before the dog killed him."

It was going to be necessary to amputate the portion of the tail where there was no skin in order to protect it from the elements. We agreed that it would be better to excise just a wee bit more tail than the injury warranted. This would enable Amigo to sport a tail comparable to that of a bobcat. Now that the cosmetic effect of a new tail length had been agreed on, George and I headed for surgery while Mr. Clark retired to the reception room to find a magazine to bide his time. George proved to be a very capable surgical assistant, and before long I was removing my surgical gloves. It was necessary to wrap the tail securely with elastic tape in order to keep the cat from chewing the stitches out. I then discon-nected the new bobtailed cat from the gas anesthetic machine, and George placed him in a recovery cage.

The hospital records were filled out and I made my way to the front room to converse with Mr. Clark. I had expected Mr. Clark to be irate about his neighbor's dog hurting Amigo but he remained rather calm. We both agreed that if the dog had gotten a firmer grip on the tail, it would have been Amigo's demise. He surprised me when he said, "That darn cat got what it deserved, but I am sure glad that dog didn't kill him." With that comment my curiosity was peaked and I had to know more. Mr. Clark was more than willing to recount the story.

The Clarks had a six-foot-high concrete block fence around their property. The neighbor on the left had a beagle-like dog and the neighbor on the other side owned a German shepherd. Amigo was a very devilish cat and walked around the top of the fence just to torment the dogs. He seemed to take delight in sitting on the fence while the dogs barked at him and tried to leap up to grab him. He felt perfectly safe on top of the fence. In fact, while all of this hullabaloo was taking place below him on the ground, Amigo sat nonchalantly on his perch and would preen himself in what he thought was complete safety.

Amigo was so efficient in antagonizing the dogs that he was becoming a nuisance in the neighborhood. The neighbors on either side were continually called by their adjoining neighbors to keep their dogs quiet. This was a huge dilemma for the Clarks. They believed their only solution was to keep Amigo in the house when either of the dogs were in their backyards. Their plan did not work very well.

Mr. Clark was barbecuing in his backyard that afternoon when he heard a cry from Amigo who was perched on top the fence watching him. He said, "I saw him jump off of the fence and race across the yard to the house. I didn't give much thought to Amigo's activities until I went into the house to get the meat to cook. It was then that noticed that Amigo was paying considerable attention to his tail. I looked closely and saw that the end of his tail had been skinned. I put Amigo into his carrier and we headed for your hospital. We are here now for your expertise."

"I think Amigo decided to watch me and he let his tail hang down over the fence. The shepherd must have made an Olympic leap and grabbed the tail, which slid out of his grasp leaving the skin behind in his mouth. He is a very lucky cat. Maybe this incident will end his tormenting the dogs." I wondered.

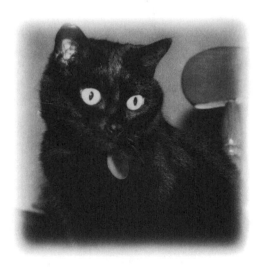

—17—

A HUGE DOG

The evening's emergencies began early. As I arrived home, Marna was waiting for me. A call had come in for a Lawndale emergency and she had already fixed a sack dinner for me. Marna mentioned that she and the boys would miss me for dinner. I would dine in the Mustang on my way to the hospital.

Before I had left the house, I had returned the call to the answering service and asked them to call the client back to tell them I was on my way to Lawndale. This sequence of phoning was always a time-saver since it allowed both the client and myself to be traveling at the same time. There was less waiting time, and if another emergency call came in, I could attend it sooner.

The hospital door had just been unlocked when the client pulled in adjacent to my Mustang. They got out of their van and opened the sliding door. Out stepped the largest Great Dane that I had ever seen. Either one of the owners could have ridden him to the hospital. All they needed was a saddle and a bridle.

Hugo had an injured foot. He was chewing at the front paw and would not let the Watkinses, his owners, look at it. Usually I request the owners to place their pet on the exam table in order for me to make a closer inspection of the injury. Hugo was too big. Four persons would be needed to lift him and at least two more to restrain him once he was placed on the exam table. We decided that rather than risk injuries to our backs it would be best to treat Hugo's injury on the floor. (I was usually reluctant to treat animals in this position—if they were vicious, it was difficult to get out of their reach in a hurry.) Hugo proved to be a great big softy. Mrs. Watkins sat on the floor and cradled Hugo's head on her lap. Mr. Watkins leaned on Hugo's body and held the injured front foot up for my inspection. All went very well despite the minor inconvenience.

Hugo had a deep cut between the pads of his foot. Stitches were required to properly take care of the injury. The lower foot was blocked with xylocaine and the surgical area was thoroughly scrubbed. At this point, Bozo was starting to get impatient. In order to decrease the time he had to be restrained in this position, I tried to hurry with the procedure. Every time I started to suture the laceration, Hugo would jerk his foot even though the anesthetic had alleviated any possibility of pain. He was now watching me and anticipating my every move. We decided that if he couldn't see what I was doing, he might hold still long enough for me to complete the surgery. I got a towel and handed it to Mrs. Watkins who then draped it over her dog's head and held it in place. It then only took a few minutes to put in the six to eight sutures that were necessary to close the wound.

I bandaged the foot and wrapped it with an elastic tape to insure that the area would be kept clean. We released Hugo and allowed him to stand. Now he really limped. His showboating was blamed on the presence of the bandage. His foot was still partially under the effects of the anesthetic so it was not painful but he insisted on carrying that foot. He gave the impression that he wanted to shake hands.

Finally I had the opportunity to ask how much Hugo weighed. He tipped the scales at two hundred eighteen pounds and stood thirty-six and one half inches at the shoulder. He was not a big dog—he was a huge dog. I stepped around the counter to complete the billing statement. Hugo rested his head on a forty-two-inch-high counter and without moving his head at all, he watched me with his eyes. The only problem was that the counter was only ten inches wide, and as he had his head stationed there, his muzzle hung over the counter and he drooled on the desk. When the owners left, I not only had to clean up the floor in the exam room, but I also had to mop up a large pool of slobber situated on the reception desk.

Not only was saliva all over the counter, but Hugo had drooled all over the calculator. I cleaned the equipment up, but could not get all the moisture out. The next time I visited this hospital, I noticed a new calcu-lator on the desk.

Marna called and said that the Clarks were trying to reach me on the Manhattan Beach line. The bandage I had placed on Amigo the taunting cat's tail had been chewed off and several stitches were missing as well. Mr. Clark met me at the hospital again. This time we were able to wrap Amigo up tightly in a blanket leaving the tail exposed. A local anesthetic block was made and the tail sutured again.

"You know, Doc," he said, "This was the best thing that ever happened to the neighborhood. Amigo lost his desire to pace the fence and irritate the dogs below. He now is content to stay on the ground in his own backyard. I think Amigo feels that he now has a new status with his bobcatlike tail. The neighbors are delighted, for the sound of dogs barking has ceased and their attitude toward each other, including us, has greatly improved. The surgery you did on Amigo's tail was definitely a good investment."

While the exam room was being cleaned up, the answering service was able to locate me. My next emergency of the evening was in Torrance and my patient was a puppy that was vomiting and had diarrhea.

Fifteen minutes later I was on location. I waited patiently for over half an hour for the clients to arrive and was about to call the answering service and have them check to see if the clients had cancelled. As I reached for the phone, a car pulled into the parking lot. They apologized for being late. Mrs. Winkler had started out the back door with the pup in her arms when the pup "barfed" all over her. It was repulsive to have that mess all over her so she went back into the house to change. It was prudent to protect the car from a future incident of this nature so as they were about to leave again, her husband returned to the house to get a towel to wrap the pup up in.

When they brought the pup into the hospital, I got a good glimpse of it and suggested that they remain holding it and not let it down on the floor. I was suspicious that the pup had some canine disease that might cause contamination and thereby expose another patient. The medical record was filled out and then the Winklers and pup were taken into the isolation ward to be examined there. Upon entry into the hospital, I had observed both a discharge from the pup's nose as well as its eyes. These symptoms that I had noted along with the clients' history of the pup having gastrointestinal problems made me very suspicious that the pup had canine distemper. The pup was examined and then put into a cage in the isolation ward. The Winklers and I retired to the front of the hospital to discuss the options that faced us.

The pup was ten weeks old. When they had purchased the pup, they were told that it had received all of the necessary vaccines and would not need further vaccination until it was a year old. I explained to them that they had been badly misinformed and showed them a vaccine record card from the hospital as an aid in explaining the normal routine vaccination program for a new dog. We discussed the disease and the dog's future. After several tears were shed, we mutually agreed that it would be best to put the pup to sleep and start over again with a healthy pet. I suggested that it may be feasible to wait a few months before getting a new dog and reminded them to be certain to take the new pup to their veterinarian as soon as possible and get it started on a proper vaccination program.

I called to tell Marna that I was coming home and found the line busy. Since I wasn't sure if Marna was talking to a friend or to the answering service, it was best to wait for a few minutes. I was biding my time waiting to call her when she called me instead. She knew I was at the Torrance hospital and told me to stay there because another case was coming in. It was a "hit-by-car" case.

A carload of tearful people arrived. "Doc, I think she is already dead," were the first words spoken as the man brought the dog through the door. His wife and several children had remained in the car. I confirmed his observation. He asked me if I could take care of his dog because he did not want his children to see it. He returned to his car and headed home. I could only guess what a gloom would prevail over that household this evening.

I took off for home and when Marna saw me pull into the driveway, she gave me a wave from the kitchen window. The boys were playing soldier in the backyard. As the eldest, Allen always played the general, the self-appointed ranking officer. His brothers had lesser ranks. Allen had been trying to organize a close-order drill but didn't appear to be too successful. There was too much insubordination. I gave each of my sons a hug and went inside.

Marna had coffee and berry pie waiting for me at the kitchen table. I went through the day's mail and she brought me up to date about her day's events. Marna asked me about mine, and from past experience, I felt it prudent to be vague. (One time the boys had asked me what I had done at the office that day and from the looks on their faces, I must have been too graphic. The next time we all sat down at the table together George said, "Don't anyone ask Dad what he did today!" I filed that comment away in my mind with the idea that I should be more careful about my mealtime conversations.)

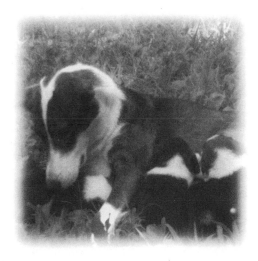

18

AN OLD-TIMER

I had a conversation with a colleague this afternoon who had just had several stitches taken in his face. While he was examining a dog, the pet's owners had become so preoccupied with what the doctor was doing that they had partially released their grip on the Labrador they were restraining. The Lab had turned on my colleague and had bitten him in the facial area. This reminder about being careful was in my thoughts as I headed for a case in Hawthorne.

This case involved a dog with a growth of some kind on the left side of the rib cage. Apparently the dog had rubbed its side against a wall or against his doghouse door. In either case, the protruding growth was abraded severely enough to cause it to hemorrhage. It needed attention of some kind. The Swensens didn't dare allow Hondo into the house because he would certainly rub his side against the furniture.

The necessary paperwork was completed and all of us entered the exam room. Hondo was a large chocolate Labrador and he growled at me when I got close to him. I thought of my colleague again. I asked the owner to lift the front end of the dog and I would assist him by lifting the tail portion where the wag is. Mr. Swensen advised me that he should lift the dog by himself. When Hondo reached the tabletop, he again growled at me and attempted to turn around and face me. The owner stated that he had complete control of his dog. Again I thought of my colleague.

The lesion on the Lab was certainly nasty in appearance. Besides rubbing his side against the wall, he had been scratching at it with his rear foot. A dressing was put on the wound and then bandaged securely with elastic tape completely around his chest. All the time a deep rumble was coming from Hondo's throat. Surgery was necessary to remove the tumor, but it could wait until morning. The Swensens were given the option of leaving Hondo overnight or bringing him in early in the morning on an empty stomach for surgery. They opted for the morning appointment. Mr. Swensen would drop him off on his way to the office.

The appointment for surgery was recorded in the schedule book and a big red star was added as a warning about the character of the Lab. The reminder from my colleague about the hazard of dealing with patients was appreciated. It was only proper for me to relay this warning about the Lab to another colleague.

It was my intent to call and ask if I could pick up anything at the grocery store on the way home. Two of the boys had been home from school the past three days with colds and sore throats. This grounded Marna at home. She seldom received help from me and this was an opportunity to help her some. The line was busy. I waited a couple of minutes and called again. The phone was still busy. I called home for the third time and Marna answered. "I have been trying to reach you but the line was busy," was her initial remark. Just then the hospital's private line rang and Marna thought that it might be the answering service's operator who had been trying to contact me at home. My wife was right. The next patient was in Lawndale, just a half-mile down the street. I had ample time to clean up the exam room and still enough time left to get a soft drink at the nearest fast-food restaurant on the way to my next patient.

As they walked into the reception room, I noticed the owners were in tears. Cuddled in a beach towel was a very old calico cat that was in terrible condition. They put their cat, wrapped in the blanket, up on the exam table. I carefully peeled back the blanket to get a better look. The cat was skin and bone. It had a bad breath with an aroma that permeated the room. While her temperature was being taken, I continued my examination. Annoyed by her fetid breath and determined to find the cause, I opened her mouth. The answer to my silent question was easy to determine, for oral cancer was prevalent not only in her mouth but had also engulfed her throat.

I looked up at the owners and they must have had the ability to read my mind. The man said, "It's hopeless, isn't it?" I remarked that the situation was very grave. They asked me to step out of the room for a few minutes. When I returned, they informed me that they had made the decision to put her to sleep. They asked to remain while I performed the task. I obliged. When all that was asked of me was accomplished, the owners remained with their pet for almost fifteen minutes.

Finally they came out carrying the towel with their calico cat inside. Since they had their cat for almost fifteen years they thought it would only be fitting to bury her at home. As I was taking care of their account, the lady remarked that their pet had had very bad breath for almost two years but they never thought about looking in her mouth. They just figured that she needed to have her teeth cleaned and they supposed that she was too old to physically handle an anesthetic. I listened quietly while they related to me about their kitty's past and how she had won the hearts of all the family members. As they were leaving, I reaffirmed them that there was nothing that could have been done and that their calico cat had lived a nice long life in a very special home. I affirmed their decision and told them that it was the most humane thing to do considering her condition. They thanked me and as they left, tears welled up in my eyes.

As they walked out the front door, I heard them say that this calico cat would be the last pet they ever owned. It was too hard emotionally for them to go through this stress again. I tried to comfort them by saying that if they once had a place in their hearts for a cat, it would be very likely that another little kitten would wedge its way into their lives. They were still standing by their car shaking their heads and shedding tears as I got into my automobile and headed for home.

I drove home slowly. I thought about the Book of Genesis in the Bible. God created all the creatures and then had Adam name all of the animals as He paraded them by. God created their life spans as well as ours and if man lives until he or she is eligible for social security, five or more cats could live to a ripe old age during that owner's lifetime.

—19—

U NEXPECTED
R ESPONSE

Marna and I were going to her sorority's annual summer banquet. It was typically a very elegant affair and we always tried to attend. Marna suggested that I not be available for any calls this evening. Her statement was, "When we go somewhere, we travel there in two cars. I am there by myself most of the time and then I have to drive home alone." Needless to say, I got the message!

I picked up the sitter for the evening and gave him instructions. In the meantime Marna left the telephone number in case he had any problems with our boys. We were off to this evening's party. We arrived at this lovely home on the peninsula, parked our car, and walked up the drive. As we walked in the front door, we were greeted by the hostess. She informed me that the answering service had been trying to reach me. I received a hostile glance from Marna but she said nothing because she knew that I had a responsibility to take these calls that came in during the night. I picked up the phone and the operator was pleased that she had been able to locate me. They found where I was from the sitter who had mistakenly given them the telephone number. The service cross-connected me and the Ralstons were now on the line. The Ralstons had an injured pet and had driven to the San Pedro hospital. They were calling from a pay phone at the corner gas station. They had left in ample time, they thought, to get to the hospital before its doors were closed for the night. Severe traffic had delayed them and when they arrived, the hospital was locked up and no

73

one was there. Their cat had a sore foot and needed medical attention. Would I please help them? I could not say, "No."

It took me a bit of time to drive to San Pedro from the peninsula hills. The Raltons brought their pet, a shorthaired yellow tabby, into the exam room. Princess was holding her right front paw up and refused to place it on the table. It was badly swollen and looked very sore. From first glance, it appeared to be a cat-bite abscess but on careful examination I could not locate any puncture wound. Her temperature was normal and thus an infection did not seem likely. I was perplexed.

A further examination was necessary. The foot was swollen from a location just above the pads down to the tip of her paw. The swollen part of her foot was cold to the touch while the part above the swollen foot felt normal. There was also a slight indentation between the swollen and normal portions of the foot. Something in the foot was acting like a tourniquet; the circulation was cut off at this point. I thought it might be something like a rubber band, and suggested this possibility to the Ralstons. Whatever was causing the problem had been on the foot long enough for the skin to overgrow it. They didn't directly say that they thought I was wrong but they gave me a skeptical look.

The Ralstons granted me permission to take an x-ray and the radiograph revealed that there was definitely something wrapped around Princess's foot. The feline was sedated and the leg prepared for investigative surgery. It did not take long to locate a rubber band. I made an incision in the skin in hopes that I could grasp the rubber band with forceps and pull it out it. Unfortunately the rubber band was friable and broke off wherever I grasped it. So it was necessary to make several incisions around the foot and remove the rubber band in pieces.

It was difficult to ascertain if the lower part of the foot was capable of restoring circulation. The rubber band had become a very effective tourniquet. My prognosis was mixed. Princess would live but her foot may have to be amputated if the circulation was not restored. The kitty was hospitalized for the night. The Ralstons were to call the doctor in the morning to see what he recommended.

The Ralstons were not surprised about the location of the rubber band on Princess's foot, for they remembered their grandchildren putting paper booties on her feet. "These booties," the Ralstons said, "were then held in place by the elastic bands. When Princess was put on the floor with her booties on, she would shake her feet in order to get them off. Finally, the booties would fly off and the children would roll with laughter. Then Princess would be shod with these paper shoes again for a repeat performance. This entertainment would go on and on until the kids tired of it. The paper boots and the rubber bands would be removed when the performance ended and Princess would run and hide. Apparently one of the bands was not noticed until now and this is the one you just found around her foot."

I got back to the party just when dessert was being served. Marna had saved a plate for me so I sat down and enjoyed that before joining the rest of our friends at the dessert table. When finished, I retired to the living room and several of the guests asked me about the case. People always seem to be interested in stories about animals. Just as I was about to relate the evening's events to the group around me, I was called to the phone again. This time it was not necessary to leave and the problem could be resolved by phone. I returned to the front room to visit with our friends.

When I finished relating about the Ralston emergency saga, several elderly ladies surrounded me to tell me of some of the stories about their pets or stories that they had heard from their friends. These same three or four ladies had a habit of cornering me at almost every party and telling me the same stories.

Marna and I had developed a code that would help me to get out of this sort of jam. If I could catch her eye, I would give her a quick cross-eyed glance and she would hurry over and rescue me. That was not the case that evening. I gave Marna the cue and she smiled back at me. I thought she missed the prearranged signal. It was repeated. The same sweet smile returned to her face. Most of the time she would dutifully come over and take my arm and say to me, "Honey, there is someone I would like you to meet" or "Would you be so kind as to get me some refreshments." Then she would lead me away from the surrounding ladies.

Tonight was different. Marna was obviously peeved at me for leaving earlier in the evening and this was her way of communicating with me that she was irritated. I couldn't help but chuckle as I again thought of that impish smile I had just seen. I now needed to extract myself from this crowd of ladies without embarrassing them or being rude. While my mind was contemplating which course to take, the hostess came over and tapped me on the shoulder and whispered to me, "You have another phone call." I now had the perfect reason to leave. I graciously excused myself and stepped into the den where the phone awaited me.

It was necessary to make another trip off the hill and I headed the car west to Redondo Beach. This case involved a cat named Creampuff that had been spayed two days earlier. It had been released this morning to the care of the owners. They realized now that something was wrong at the site of the incision. "The cat's guts are coming out," was the Nordoffs' comment. I surmised that the problem was a dehiscence (when some of the skin sutures come out and some of the underlying tissue is visible). But it was necessary to see the cat to be certain that it was not something more serious.

The Nordoffs were extremely agitated. The doctor had told them that it was a routine surgery and everything would be okay. But, obviously, everything was not okay! Creampuff had chewed out several sutures and there was some underlying tissue exposed. The owners again reminded me that her insides were coming out. This was not the case, but I understood why they thought that.

My examination revealed that a dehiscence had occurred. I explained to the Nordoffs that there was another layer of stitches that were still retaining the contents of the abdominal cavity. But they were so upset that it was very difficult to communicate with them. My most grueling task of the evening was to calm them down.

I would have preferred to bandage Creampuff's abdomen and let the doctor in the morning handle this case. But something needed to be done immediately to make the clients happy. Kitty was hooked up to the gas anesthetic machine and the sutures replaced. In order to be certain that Creampuff would not chew out her stitches as before, I placed a secure elastic bandage around her middle. I then put Creampuff in a cage and went out to the front room where the Nordoffs were waiting. I informed them that she could not be discharged until she recovered from the anesthetic so it would be necessary keep her overnight.

The Nordoffs asked to see their cat before they left, so they came to the ward to take a glimpse. When Mrs. Nordoff saw her kitty, she asked, "Does she really have to have that bandage around her?" I explained that sometimes we bandage the suture area to insure that the pet will not pay attention to the surgery. Mrs. Nordoff continued by saying that when they had picked Creampuff up the morning after surgery, she had a bandage on just like the one she had on now. "Did she chew it off?" I asked. "No, Doctor," was the reply, "I took it off because it annoyed her."

That greatly disturbed me. After regaining my composure, I shared with them that when bandages are put on a pet, they are put on for a purpose. I went on to say that they should always consult the doctor before making any changes. A spirited discussion occurred between the owners. Mr. Nordoff reprimanded his wife for taking the bandage off. He even inferred she was stupid for removing it. I kept quiet.

As the lively discussion continued between the Nordoffs, I suggested we return to the front of the hospital to carry on our conversation so that the other pets in the ward would not be disturbed. I told them that in the morning the doctor would review the night's cases and it would be best to give him a call at that time to check up on Creampuff. As they started out the door they were still mumbling to each other. Neither one of them was happy.

Before returning to the party, I thought it would be prudent to swing by the San Pedro hospital and check on the Ralston cat. Princess was sitting up in her cage, licking her injured paw. The paw felt warm again and there was some fresh blood around the nails of the foot. I phoned the Ralstons to give them an update. I apologized for the late call and they said that they had not retired yet. I told them the good news: Princess looked as if she would not be a three-legged cat. They thanked me for taking the time to phone and said they would sleep much better now.

It was well past time for the party to be over so I called our house to see if Marna was there. She answered the phone. Another guest had brought her home, but she was waiting for me to come and take the sitter home. She could not do it because she did not want to leave the boys alone. When would I be home?

Fifteen minutes later I arrived home. The sitter was taken home, and when I stepped through the back door, Marna immediately reminded me that she was at the party alone almost the entire evening. I didn't help matters any when I told her that I did take her to the party and that she didn't drive home alone. It would have been much better for me to have remained silent—my remarks did not set well with Marna. Thankfully she spoke to me the following morning.

—20—

MONKEY BUSINESS

I just put down the telephone. The answering service had wanted to know if I would be willing to treat a rhesus monkey. I explained to them that I was not familiar with the treatment of exotic animals and recommended they call another veterinarian in the area who was known to have considerable skill in the treatments of primates. The day's mail was beckoning for my attention so I returned to my chair in the family room to take care of that matter. The phone rang again. The operator had the same party on the line that had called a few minutes ago. The doctor that I had recommended to take the service call was not available. The owner desired to consult me so I obliged—after all, I only had to talk on the phone.

The owner's complaint was that their monkey, Oscar, had hives and was very uncomfortable. In fact, the rhesus was scratching himself so much, she felt that he might abrade himself with his nails. I explained to her that I was not very familiar with the treatment of primates. She remarked, "Good gosh, Doctor, he has hives and all he needs is an injection of an antihistamine." If her diagnosis was correct, I told her that her recommendation for resolving the problem was correct. I agreed to meet her at the Lawndale hospital. As I was on my way, I had mixed emotions about the case. I was not experienced in handling monkeys and there would be no assistants there to assist me. Only the owner would be present, although she had sounded capable over the phone. Only time would tell if this monkey was to be a problem case. Why wasn't her regular veterinarian available? Was it because he had previous undesirable experiences with his patient or was he just out of town? I had twenty minutes for all these questions to traverse my mind before I arrived at the hospital.

The monkey was brought into the hospital in a large cage. I was glad and ushered the client into the exam room and closed the door. I took the monkey's temperature and examined its skin. Hives were present and I agreed with the lady that this skin condition had all of the earmarks of an allergic reaction. I filled the syringe with the proper dosage of the antihistamine, benedryl. The entire procedure was closely monitored by the rhesus. I obtained cotton from the supply jar, saturated it with alcohol, and dabbed it on the skin where I intended to inject the medicine.

Unknowingly, I had pushed the calamity button. All heck broke lose. The rhesus bit its owner on the hand and she released her grip on her pet. Now there was an unrestrained monkey sashaying around the room. Thank goodness I had the foresight to close the door before allowing the pet out of its cage. The exam room was much larger than his cage and it gave him a great opportunity to stretch out and exercise. Full advantage of this freedom was taken. Several laps were taken around the room and nothing in the room proved to be a barrier; he hurdled the chair and table whenever needed. He even decided that some of the glass supply jars full of cotton and sponges would look better on the floor. He completed his "endurance run" on top of the refrigerator, raising his upper lip at both of us and surveying the damage he had done.

The monkey seemed happy to just stay where he was and stare at us. While he remained quiet, I checked the owner's hand. There did not appear to be any significant damage even though it was very painful. The next task was to get the troublemaker off the refrigerator and back on the table where he could be treated. The owner said that there was no way the monkey would come down while I was in the room because he was now frightened of me. Underneath, I too was frightened of this thirty-pound dynamo. I was more than happy to oblige her request and so I left the room. Shortly, the exam room door opened, and the owner peeked out and asked for a broom and a dustpan which I gladly provided. "It may take Oscar ten or fifteen minutes more to regain his composure," was her comment. I decided to regain my own composure over a cup of coffee during this hiatus.

The fifteen minutes stretched into almost a half-hour before I was invited to return to the exam room. The room had been cleaned up and Oscar was on the table waiting to be treated. Another syringe was filled with antihistamine and I approached my opponent with extra caution. Oscar's head was held securely this time so he could not bite anyone, especially me.

As I began to administer the injection in the back part of his rear leg, he reached back between his hind legs and tried to grab the syringe out of my hand. This scenario was repeated several times. Finally I won the battle and the medicine was now deep in the muscle of Oscar's rear leg. The rhesus was deposited in his cage and the door securely latched. It was a relief to know that I had won the final engagement.

Oscar was carried out to the car and the owner returned to pick up her prescription. I sent home some teledron capsules that had time-relief granules in them so she could sprinkle some of the medicine on Oscar's food. I could not envision the owner giving anything orally to her pet, although it did not appear to me that the rhesus was dangerous. (Animals have a much better sense of smell than humans and I think that he may have perceived the scent of some other pet in the exam room and become terrified.) When monkey, owner, and car pulled out of the parking lot, I gave a sigh of relief. Another cup of coffee settled my nerves before it was time for me to head home.

On my way home I realized how thankful I was that my own practice was almost 100 percent canine and feline. The lights were still on in the boys' rooms as I approached the house. I gave Marna a brief overview of my night's events, but she soon stopped me because she wanted me to share the experience with my sons.

We had the boys come out to the family room in their pajamas and gather around the fireplace. Marna provided freshly baked cookies and hot apple cider as the boys sat on cushions around the room. I asked Albert to get up so he could get his teddy bear from his room. That evening's entertainment was an animated feature about a silly veterinarian and a wild monkey.

The teddy bear was now the monkey, the coffee table the exam table, and the television the refrigerator. A pencil became a syringe. I used the teddy bear to demonstrate my night's experience. When I arrived at the exam room counter with the frightened teddy, I looked for something to throw on the floor. Marna cautioned me not to be too dramatic. By the time the wild monkey rendition reached the curtain call, the boys were all laughing and Marna was in tears. All three of the boys were hard to tuck in that night due to the exciting drama. George even asked if it really happened. I vowed to refer any primate emergencies in the future.

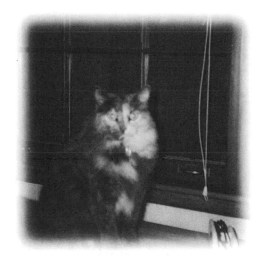

─21─

HIDE-AND-SEEK

It was raining outside this Sunday afternoon and the boys were confined to the house. My sons had unlimited energy and were playing soldier by running through the house and having a brief skirmish at each doorway. They were making sounds like bombs and grenades going off. This normally was fine. But this time I was trying to converse with the service on the telephone. Two calls were in the mill—both from the Torrance hospital. Finally I asked Marna to corral the boys in the other room so I could hear the specifics concerning the cases.

I talked to the first client. Her name was Pat Duprey. She stated that she had sprayed something on her cat's face and now her cat couldn't open its eyes. Could I meet her at the hospital right away as she was about to leave on a trip? I told her that I would be at the hospital in fifteen minutes. She would be there waiting for me. The second call was from an elderly lady who had made the decision to put her pet to sleep. I scheduled this for forty-five minutes after the first call. It was infrequent that two calls would come in at the same time for the same hospital.

When I arrived at the hospital, Miss Duprey was waiting at the door. She was holding a cat carrier and appeared to be in a hurry. As I unlocked the door, I noticed that she was in uniform. I commented that she must be a United Airline stewardess. She corrected me by saying that she was a "flight attendant" of that airline.

As we entered the exam room, she said, "Doctor, I am in a terrible rush. I have a flight to catch. I did a stupid thing. Daphne walked up to

82

me while I was spraying an aerosol foot powder on my feet. I was being cute and gave her a puff of it in her face. I didn't realize that it would cause an irritation to her eyes until I was ready to leave for the airport. Daphne was in the kitchen with her eyes closed and tears streaming down her face. Doctor, I can't wait. Here is the can of spray I used. Daphne is in the carrier and here is a fifty-dollar deposit. I'm out of here. I'll call from New York in the morning to check on her. Do whatever needs to be done. Bye now."

It felt like a whirlwind had just passed through the room. I took the carrier into the treatment room and removed Daphne. I was now gazing at a beautiful silver Persian cat that was very well groomed. Her eyes were still tightly closed and tearing. The inside fur of each of her forepaws was wet as she had tried in vain to wipe whatever was bothering her out of her eyes. The eyes were rinsed with a saline solution and ointment was applied to them for comfort. Her face and feet still contained a residue from the spray so I dutifully washed them to remove any possibility of the chemicals in the spray getting into her eyes again. Even after spot-bathing her, the smell of the spray persisted so I put a leash on her and plunged her into the bathtub. She had just been lathered up when my next client arrived. I decided to let her soak. I securely tied the leash to the tub's faucet while I went to the front of the hospital and took care of the new arrivals.

Mrs. Tolson was sitting there with her pet, a West Highland terrier. I remembered both she and her dog because I had treated the Westie almost three years ago at this very hospital during the day practice. Searching through the files, the Westie's card was located under the owner's name, Martha and David Tolson. The dog's name was Bingo. According to the records, Bingo had lived fourteen summers. He was in very poor physical condition. He had lost a lot of weight and Mrs. Tolson said that he had difficulty getting up and down, and when he did get up, he had difficulty walking. Mrs. Tolson alerted me by saying, "I am eighty-two now and it is very difficult for me to carry Bingo when he has to go outside to take care of his chores." I commented that according to the hospital records, she had not been in for several years. "I haven't been able to drive for the past ten years and when my husband, David, died three years ago, I became housebound. After David left, Bingo would follow me around the house. I talked to him all the time. I would say, 'Bingo, let's go make the bed' and he would follow me into the bedroom while I performed that task. Then I would say, 'Bingo, let's go have a cookie,' and he would follow me into the kitchen for his treat. Bingo followed me everywhere and he was a wonderful companion. Now he can't get around and he is too much for me to carry around at my age. I would like to wait here while you take care of him."

Cradling Bingo in my arms, I retired to the back of the hospital to fulfill her request. When I returned to the reception room, Martha was sitting in a chair in a daze staring out through the front window. Another chair was pulled up and I sat down beside her in an attempt to render some comfort. At this point, she lost her composure and began crying. I was afraid that she was going to faint so I retreated to the other room and brought her a glass of water. For several minutes we just sat there in silence. It was necessary to help her out to her taxi that was still waiting for her. As she got into the cab, she turned to me and said, "You know, Doctor, I am completely alone now. David and I were never blessed with children and now I have outlived everyone else in the family." Tears were welling up in my eyes as I gave her a hug and said good-bye to her for the last time.

When I got inside, I returned to the grooming room to complete Daphne's bath. She wasn't in the bathtub. The only indication that she had been there was the severed piece of nylon leash which was hanging limp from the faucet. When any animal escapes within a hospital, the first thing I do is to immediately shut every door. This confines them to any room in which they may have sought refuge. The second job is to locate them. I began my search. Every room was checked. My effort was futile. She had to be in the hospital somewhere since there was no opportunity for her to exit the premises. Again I searched and this time with more diligence. I went through each room searching in, behind, and under anything that may have shielded her from my previous effort to locate her. Leaning against the wall, I made an effort to reason like a cat. She was very small and felines always feel more secure in dark places since they can see just as well there as in bright places. All of the cupboards and cabinets had been closed so that possibility was scratched from the list. Then I remembered closing the storeroom door which I had left open when I got the shampoo. The storage room needed a more thorough inspection. On the lower shelf there was a stack of newspapers. On the top sheet of paper were several water spots indicating to me that Daphne had been here. I reached behind the stack and felt wet fur. Success at last!

I put Daphne back in the tub for the completion of her bath. A good toweling followed. I again applied medicine to her eyes, and then deposited her into the drying cage. While she was drying, I cleaned the hospital so it would be ready for the morning shift. I was part of that shift and didn't want to hear any static from the staff when they arrived.

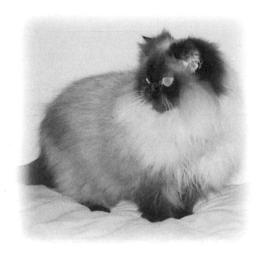

— 22 —

THE TROPHY

It was now mid-June. The rain had stopped. Spring was behind us and the sun was casting its rays down on the earth in earnest. This course of nature causes the grass to turn brown and the foxtails to become a nuisance to animals, for now they had reached their maturity. (Foxtails are a big problem for the pet population and represent a good source of income for veterinarians. Besides being found in their natural places in the fields, they can be found in many other places. They often appear in dog's feet, in their ears, eyes and nose, in tonsillar crypts, and even in their genitalia. I make many trips to various hospitals to remove these undesirable foreign body pests during the summer months.)

I had the privilege of speaking to a Scotswoman that day. The service quickly turned the conversation over to me because she was very hard to understand. She had a dog that was sneezing profusely and shaking its head. To me, it sounded as if the dog had a foxtail in its nares. She desired that her dog have medical attention but objected to the emergency fee. After some discussion, she agreed to meet me at the hospital in spite of the charges that had been quoted.

We met at the Palos Verdes hospital. She brought in a Border collie that was in considerable distress. Her dog was sneezing blood by now. I hurriedly escorted the two of them into the exam room so that I would not have blood to clean up in the reception room. I lifted her dog up on the exam table for her to hold. She was such a petite lady that there was no way she was going to be able to hold a forty-pound dog. I informed her that it would be necessary to sedate her dog in order to perform a nasal examination. She asked, "How much will that cost?" I quoted the hospital's fee and she told me that it cost too much. "Why don't you get one of your assistants to hold my dog?" was her next question. I explained that I was the only person at the hospital at that time of day and that it would cost about the same if I had to call someone at home to come down and lend a hand. Even if one of my assistants was here, it may still be necessary to sedate her dog in order to hold it steady enough to check its nose.

Finally she agreed to do the exam my way. I sedated her Border collie with surital and added a little demerol to the intravenous injection to decrease the sneezing reflex. Then an endotracheal tube was placed in the trachea so her dog's respirations would be vented to the end of the tube. This kept her humid respired air from fogging up the lens on my otoscope. The foxtail was located immediately. Using a pair of alligator forceps, I grasped the awns of the foxtail and extracted the entire weed from the right nostril. I showed Mrs. Mac Cool the trophy. She was very happy that I had found the cause of her dog's sneezing episode but she still showed displeasure concerning the quoted fee. She said, "I know what all of you veterinarians do on your days off. You fly around over the city and look for vacant lots to scatter all of these foxytail seeds so you can make more money."

I could not help but chuckle to myself about her remarks. I decided to remain silent as it was not necessary to continue the discussion. She opened her purse to settle her account and all I could see was a field of greenbacks. Her purse was loaded with money. She paid me in cash rather grudgingly. I carried her pet out to her car and gave her instructions for its aftercare. She backed the car around as I stood there watching her head for the road. As she passed me, she rolled down the car window and said, "Thank you, young man." She had a soft spot in her heart after all.

The trip up the coast was pleasant. The sun was shining brightly and the beach was swarming with bathers. I had to slow down several times to allow surfers with their boards to cross the street. There were several routes that I could take to get to Hermosa Beach, but on a nice day I wanted to see more than blacktop and traffic signs. I chose the scenic route along the coast.

My next case was a dog that had a sore front foot. I suspected that this would be another foxtail case for me this day. I guessed incorrectly as it proved to be a nail problem instead. The dewclaw nail had grown so long that it had curled around like a bighorn sheep's horn and embedded itself in the fleshy part of the foot. The foot was very sore—as the nail grows it penetrates deeper. Bacteria and the like are on the nails and these organisms are deposited under the skin causing a severe infection. In all, I was looking at a very inflamed foot.

It did not take long to cut the nail in two and then to remove the portion that had penetrated the flesh. The owner could not understand how this could happen. He said, "Skippy runs all over the place. I thought his nails would be constantly ground down by all of his activity." The injured foot had already been bandaged, so I demonstrated with the opposite foot. I pointed to the dewclaw pad and nail. "It never touches the ground when he is walking or running so there is no opportunity for it to be sanded down by the street or sidewalk." "By golly, I never realized that!" he exclaimed.

The remainder of Rusty's nails were trimmed to avoid future calamities. I felt that the owner never took time to look at his dog's feet. (Many owners feed and pat their pets but don't pay any other attention to them until their pet does something to attract their attention.)

My last case of the evening was in Hawthorne so I turned my car east away from the beautiful sunset. Occasional views of the setting sun were noticed in the rearview mirror. I could still appreciate the effects of the sunset in the pink clouds overhead.

The Wallaces were bringing in Ginger, their Irish setter, who had been treated many times for a persistent skin problem. The dog had an odor that was so bad that it could drive anyone out of the room. It was not initially noticed as they entered the hospital, but it did not take long before the odor permeated the front room. This was the second or third time I had seen Ginger about her skin, as I was on duty at this location on Mondays.

Ginger needed to be on medication continually to control her flaky skin and the alopecia that accompanied the problem. Regular medicated baths had previously been prescribed as a necessity for the improvement of the skin. Both her skin and hair problems could have been brought under control if she had been given a better diet. We had bathed her many times at the hospital and sent home bottles of shampoo for the owners to use on her. The shampoo containers were never opened. Medication had been dispensed but the prescription never refilled. A suitable diet had been recommended but never implemented. I was more than frustrated with the owners, for they seemed so indifferent about the health and well-being of Ginger. I even explained to the owner that when buying dog food, you get what you pay for. If you feed a dog inexpensive food then you will require veterinary services more often.

It was my intention to lay all of the cards on the table at one time. There was a risk that I would lose a client or rather the hospital would. The owners had been spending a lot of money on their pet and Ginger's skin looked the same or worse every time it was seen. Her condition reflected neglect. The Wallaces probably had enough shampoo at home to open a pet shop. I intended to be abrupt and to the point with them. I was just that. I reprimanded them for the quality of care they were providing Ginger. Changes were necessary. I even emphasized that if they would spend more money for better quality dog food, they would spend much less money for veterinary care.

I again put Ginger on a high protein diet. I gave her a steroid injection of vetalog for the immediate relief of the pruritis and some tablets of the same product were sent home to extend the level of the injection. I could not bathe her this evening but I sent shampoo home to be certain that they would have the type that I wanted them to use.

A deal was cut with the Wallaces. If Ginger did not show a marked improvement in thirty days, I would refund all of their expenses that they had incurred this evening. They smiled and agreed to accept the challenge.

—23—

EYE PROBLEM

Greta always greeted me at the yard gate or the back door of the house whenever I arrived home. She was basically my dog, but she accepted attention from all members of the family—especially when a nutritional treat was in the offering. Greta also enjoyed riding in the car. If Marna or I jingled our car keys, she would impatiently wait and prance at the exit door anxiously awaiting an invitation to join us on our trip. She preferred the seat next to the driver and would sit there as any attentive adult would. She missed nothing and every movement caught her eye. I only wish that she could communicate with me, as she certainly was more observant of her surroundings than I.

This Saturday she begged to go with me and almost crowded me out of the way as I tried to open the back door. Her impatient waiting at the door relayed to me her desire to join me on this trip to the hospital.

I glanced at the fuel indicator on the car. I had acquired a habit of doing this since I had run out of gas already twice this year. My gas tank was dangerously low so I pulled into my regular station to fill the tank of the Mustang. As soon as I left the driver's seat to leave a deposit for the gasoline, Greta moved over into the warm seat that I had just vacated. As the tank was being filled, a customer noted our German shorthair sitting in the driver's seat and jokingly said, "Do you allow your dog to drive?" Without batting an eye, I said, "She has a license!" The other customer had meant driver's license and I deliberately referred to a rabies license. I nudged Greta over as I got into the Mustang. I looked in the rearview mirror as I pulled out and noted that the customer was looking our way and had a rather perplexed expression on his face.

At the hospital, Greta immediately resumed her position behind the wheel and became my watchdog. The Brunners brought in Omar, their tabby cat, who had an injured eye. I usually see eye cases in very early stages, for pet owners can immediately relate to ocular injuries. Omar had come into the house that morning squinting with his right eye. He had been out all night, and after being let into the house was not his old self. The eye was definitely bothering him. Food was sniffed at and not eaten. His special cushion had not been occupied. He hid himself under the owners' bed where it was dark. His general demeanor was one of solitude, and that was completely out of character for Omar. During the morning, Omar remained in self-imposed exile. When he was brought out from under the bed and placed by his food dish, he would smell it and then hustle back to his sanctuary under the bed. When Omar continued to rub the eye, the Brunners decided that Omar's eye needed attention.

I selected the topical eye anesthetic, ophthaine. A couple of drops in the eye would render the eye insensitive to my examination. The eyelids were deflected so I could get a clear view of the cornea. An abrasion on the cornea was evident. My observation was confirmed by using a fleuroscene strip that enabled the corneal abrasion to become more evident—a corneal ulcer was present. It was a large ulcer and undoubtedly very uncomfortable to Omar whenever he blinked. This is the reason he had sought a dark place in which to hide.

It would be necessary to protect the eye from the irritation of light as well as self-inflicted damage. I discussed with the Brunners the need of a conjunctival flap. (The conjunctiva is reflected over the cornea and sutured in place, thus protecting the cornea with a layer of tissue.) This flap would remain in place for about ten days, and medication would have to be put in the eye five or six times daily.

I proceeded with surgery with the Brunners' permission. Omar stayed the night and all day Sunday as well. Between the staff and me, the medication was applied every four hours. We alternated the medication—atropine was given the first time, and polymyxin-B the next time. When the conjunctiva had been sutured to cover the eye, one stitch had been left out to provide a small gap so that the medication could be applied properly.

When I stopped by late Sunday evening, one-eyed Omar was looking out of his cage at me begging for personal attention. His food dish was empty. But he did not appreciate it when I administered the eye medication. However, he purred when I petted him as I returned him to his cage.

Greta was impatiently waiting for my return. I took her for a quick walk in one of the hospital's runs, then jingled my keys, and she headed for the front door. Before I left the hospital, I had a feeling that it would be best to call home and check with Marna. I had neglected to tell her to which hospital I was going. She informed me that I did have a call. I called that answering service to find out more about the call and which hospital line it had come in on. They actually had two calls for me—one at Hermosa Beach and another at Torrance.

The first call I was able to resolve over the phone. It concerned mostly questions and predictions. Questions I handled as best as possible on the phone. Predictions were postponed until the patient could be examined, for it was in the best interest of all concerned not to pin down the referring veterinarian with a diagnoses and/or a solution. It would be improper to tell the doctor what to do even if I had seen the case. Patient cases change overnight as do medical decisions. I never would want a client to tell a doctor that I indicated the case should be treated in a specific manner.

The emergency at the Torrance hospital needed attention. A cat had some cuts on its feet and blood was being tracked throughout her house. Mrs. Lambert brought in an Abyssinian cat that she had wrapped in a terry cloth towel and then stuffed into a portable cage.

Mrs. Lambert told me about her escapade with Sinbad. In order for me to understand what happened, it was necessary for her to describe the circumstances that led up to the catastrophe.

For some time, Mrs. Lambert had noticed that dust was removed in places on the beams on her vaulted ceiling in the living room. She thought nothing of it. Later, she caught Sinbad climbing up the drapes and sitting on the wooden valance. From the valance he could reach the first beam—from there he could jump from beam to beam as only four feet separated them. That evening she had taken appetizers to a party and returned with a tray full of dishes. At the front door, she carefully balanced the tray on one hand as waiters commonly do, unlocked the front door, and stepped into the front room. As she was taking the key out of the lock, Sinbad jumped from the beam onto the tray. Tray, leftover edibles, dishes, and Sinbad crashed to the floor. The mess was not her concern at this time. Sinbad was the problem.

"As soon as Sinbad hit the floor, he took off for the bedroom for refuge. I thought it was great that he left, for now he would not be in the way while I cleaned up. When I began to pick up the large pieces of broken glass, I noticed bloody cat tracks on both the hardwood floor and on the carpet. I tracked Sinbad down the hall and into the bedroom. There he was—on the bed licking his cut feet. I bundled him up in a towel and called the hospital."

The injury was not severe. All four feet required pressure bandages to stop the hemorrhaging. No sutures were required. I administered penicillin intramuscularly as a precaution to avoid infection. He was then returned to his cage. He did not know which foot to pay attention to as all four feet were taped up, so he just tucked his front feet under him and curled up in the corner of his cage.

Mrs. Lambert was not excited about returning to her house and cleaning up the mess. She asked me how it would be most practical to avoid a recurrence. Since the only access Sinbad had to get up on the beams was the drapes, and the only way he could climb the drapes were with front claws, I suggested that she have surgery done to remove the claws. I recommended that she discuss this surgery with her regular veterinarian.

Mrs. Lambert and I left the hospital at the same time. I carried Sinbad out in his cage and put him into the backseat of her car. Greta was watching me carefully from the Mustang. She greeted me with enthusiasm as I got in the car. Greta sniffed me carefully to see what strange pet I had associated with. I had brought out a dog biscuit from the hospital and placed it in my shirt pocket. She finally located it and waited patiently for me to hand it to her. She lay down on the seat and munched it on the way home.

24

THE PORCUPINE

Clients desire to visit their regular veterinary hospital rather than visit a new one when they are traveling. This was the case early Sunday morning. The Collinses had taken their five- month-old Boxer, Chip, on a camping trip in the Sierra Mountains.

I arrived at the hospital almost an hour before the Collinses. After they had called, they decided to break camp now rather than having to return to the mountains later in the day to perform the same task.

Mr. Collins said, "Chip loves the fresh smell of mountain air and the new terrain. He spent all day Saturday investigating every rock, stream, and tree he could find. At night he was exhausted and crashed in our tent and slept until early hours of this morning. At daybreak he nuzzled me and wanted to go outside the tent for a run. We let him out. We watched him from the tent flap. With his nose to the ground, he circled the tent and as he dropped out of sight behind the picnic table, he gave a yelp and headed back to the tent. Porcupine quills were protruding from his muzzle and tongue. He was in anguish." At five months of age, Chip was still a student. He still had a lot to learn about Mother Nature and her inhabitants.

The Collinses had been very wise in not trying to pull out any of the quills, for frequently they break off in the attempt. (Porcupine quills have minute barbs on them and are very difficult to extract from tissue. If the quills do break off, the retained part needs to be surgically dissected from the tissue.)

Chip was in extreme pain and was pawing at his face and whining in discomfort. In doing this, some of the quills had been broken at the surface of his skin. I sedated Chip with surital and connected him to the metafane gas anesthetic machine. He had nine quills in him. Seven were easily removed but two had broken off—one in his tongue and one in his lip. Incisions were made alongside each of these two retained quills until enough quill was visible to enable me to grasp it with forceps. Then with gentle retraction, each quill came free. No sutures would be required for closure. The cheek and the tongue would be sore for some time, but a young dog will soon heal. I was certain that Chip would long remember this camping experience.

The Collinses were glad that Chip had not encountered a skunk. A skunk would have presented a much different problem for the Collins family. It would have only been uncomfortable for Chip. The Collins family was debating this issue as they pulled out of the parking lot.

Church was over and my family was at home when I returned. The boys had requested waffles, and Marna was getting the ingredients out of the cupboard when she realized that she had no Bisquick. She asked me to toodle down to the nearest market and purchase some. I came up with a better idea. Why not all of us go out for brunch and get waffles. Before I had concluded my suggestion, Marna was putting items back into the cupboard, and the boys were heading for the car. No one said that it was a good idea, but I could tell by their actions that they were responding in a positive manner.

We had to wait for a half-hour to be seated so I felt I should contact the services and let them know my location. Halfway through brunch, the waitress informed me of a telephone call. It was not a "right now" emergency, but one that needed to be seen. I try not to divulge too much about cases at the table, so when I returned, Marna and the boys were told that I planned to stop by the Torrance hospital on my way home.

The Fillmores had a basset hound, Archie, that was vomiting intermittently. The problem appeared to be getting worse. When they saw the five of us pile out of the car, they were very apologetic for disturbing my time with my family. However, they were very appreciative of my availability.

It took two of us to place Archie on the exam table. No sooner had he placed his feet on the table, than dry heaves occurred. His temperature was normal, and his chest and abdomen both sounded normal. I then proceeded to palpate his abdomen, and a hard object about the size of a golf ball was felt in his stomach.

We carefully stretched Archie on his side and took both a dorsoventral and a lateral radiograph. He was put on the floor while I spent a few minutes in the darkroom developing the film. We looked at the radiograph together and saw a beautiful outline of a pocket watch. Neither of the Fillmores could understand what they now were viewing. Even Marna and the boys came in for a look at the film. The diagnosis was unanimous.

Archie was given an anesthetic and taken into surgery. After he was connected to the anesthetic machine, he was scrubbed and otherwise prepared for surgery. Allen became my assistant while Marna and my younger two sons visited with the Fillmores in the reception room. We commenced with the gastrotomy. Forty-five minutes later, Allen and I went out to the reception room with our prize. As we opened the door, Mr. Fillmore asked me what time was on the pocket watch. I showed him a large fish weight that had a wire at the top making its silhouette look like a pocket watch.

We figured the weight must have smelled like fish or bait of some kind. Archie had picked it up as he was licking it off, and accidentally swallowed it. This rendition was very plausible. It was very difficult for the Fillmores to understand because neither of them fished or had any fishing gear around the premises. How or where Archie acquired this fish weight was beyond their comprehension.

Archie was hospitalized and the Fillmores left for home. The five of us worked together to clean the hospital, and then, we too, headed for home. On the way, I compensated the boys and Marna for the interruption and stopped at the corner ice cream parlor for cones. We arrived home and the boys jumped out of the car jostling George, causing him to drop the ice cream from his cone. He was upset, but he decided to give Greta a treat. Greta was more than willing to share "cone day" with her family.

I wasn't home long. Foxtail season was still in session. The number of cases gradually diminished yearly as more vacant lots were converted to building sites. In these vacant fields, wild oats thrived, and were the nemesis of pets that frequently used these locations for playgrounds. Foxtails, the seeds of wild oats, have a habit of attaching themselves to the coat of animals, and then migrating into more strategic locations.

Late that afternoon, I was on my way to treat a coughing dog. Pepe, a well-groomed white poodle, had been coughing for two days. The owners, themselves, had experienced sore throats and thought possibly that Pepe had acquired a cough and a sore throat from them. Pepe had a mild fever, and when I examined his throat, it was very red and swollen. I allowed the information given by the clients to influence my diagnosis. All Pepe had was a sore throat, and I treated him accordingly.

As I was lifting him from the exam table, I noticed bloodstained whiskers. I realized that just coughing usually does not cause the throat to bleed. I recalled reading in *The Veterinary Journal* about a dog with foxtails embedded in its throat. Pepe was still in my arms, so I placed him back on the table, and decided to be more thorough in my examination. I opened his mouth again. I grasped his tongue and pulled it forward to obtain a better view of his throat. On the left side a localized swelling was visible.

With permission, Pepe was given a short-acting anesthetic of surital. An oral speculum was used to keep his mouth open and free both of my hands. The Maynards were instructed to hold Pepe's head in direct line with the spotlight to enhance my vision. Carefully, I probed the left tonsillar crypt, and fortunately was able to locate the awn of a foxtail. The awn was grasped and with careful teasing, the entire foxtail was extracted.

I had already given medication for the sore throat, so no further treatment was necessary. A mixture of honey and warm water was advised. It was to be given, as needed, to soothe Pepe's throat whenever he coughed.

On my drive home, I realized that I had now located one more place on a pet's body that was not safe from a foxtail invasion.

Marna and I were enjoying a late cup of coffee as we visited. It was almost midnight when the phone rang, and the answering service asked me to talk to the Watsons, who owned a nursing bitch named Christy. Christy had a very swollen breast—it was red and sore, and they suspected an infection. They had planned to wait until morning, but it was bothering her so much, she would not allow any of her pups to nurse. They were also afraid that if the pups did nurse, they might get sick, and then they would have a real problem on their hands. I concurred with their reasoning and agreed to meet them at the hospital.

The Watsons arrived with their Christy, a mixed cockapoo, who had an enlarged and very hard thoracic breast. The breast was so swollen that it appeared it might burst at any moment. The Watsons helped by gently holding her while I administered surital in her vein. I then carried Christy into the treatment room while her owners returned to the reception room to wait.

A small incision was made at one edge of the swollen breast, and at least two cups of purulent matter flowed out into an abscess pan. Floating in the midst of all of the discharge was a foxtail. The abscess area was flushed with a saline solution. I applied an antibiotic ointment called panalog to the lesion. It was then that I noted a puddle of water by her left front foot. No solution had been spilt there, and the table was not wet between the foot and the area where I had lavaged the breast.

I was puzzled. I checked Christy's foot, and moisture was present between her toes. I noted a lesion in that same location. I inserted a fifty-milliliter syringe full of saline solution into the foot lesion, and moisture appeared in the breast area. I now realized how the foxtail had gained access to the mammary tissue. The origin of entry was the foot, and the foxtail had migrated to the breast and then an abscess had formed.

Now that the infection had been treated and the source of the problem had been removed, healing should rapidly occur. In order to allow the pups to nurse and to keep them away from the discharge, so they would not get sick, I suggested to the Watsons that they keep the pups from nursing on the thoracic breasts. To accomplish this, I asked them to get a child's T-shirt and put it over Christy's head. Then I asked them to pull Christy's legs through the arms and with the elastic tape I was giving them, to tape the shirttail to her body. This would insure that the pups would not get to the infected breast. It would be necessary to roll up the shirttail and treat the infection with the panalog ointment that I was dispensing. After each treatment, the shirt would need to be retaped to her body.

As I was driving home, I realized that on that day I had become personally aware of two more locations where foxtails can cause problems on a pet. It was almost two in the morning when I arrived home. I found Marna curled up in my leather chair fast asleep with a book on her lap.

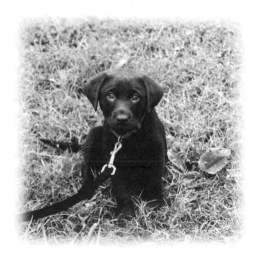

— 25 —

IN-HOUSE PICNIC

Marna had planned the day well in advance. A picnic had been scheduled. It was a holiday. I did not have to work at my daytime practice, and all three of the boys would be home from school. We would have the day to ourselves! The likelihood of having any emergencies was nil, for most of my colleagues would be home and covering for their own practices. The only concern we had was the weather. Ominous-looking clouds were beginning to appear in the northwest. When we first got up in the morning, Marna said the sky was clear as she brought in the newspaper. The sun had been shining and inclement weather was nowhere in sight. The five of us shrugged off the possibility of rain and proceeded with our plans.

When I arrived in the kitchen, Marna was already selecting items for the picnic basket. I had a quick cup of coffee and a rapid peruse of the newspaper before I left to make my rounds at both Redondo Beach and Torrance. I wanted to leave early, do my treatments, and return before the boys were in motion.

Five animals needed my attention at Redondo Beach and I was on my way in the Mustang to Torrance within an hour. I was greeted at the glass front door by a dog looking at me as I approached. This was not a good start for me there as animals were supposed to be caged at all times. This mixed shepherd was more than glad to see someone and this morning that someone was me. I got into the hospital without my "greeter" escaping. I encouraged him to follow me. He pranced along behind me, and appeared to be happy to have company after being alone all night.

There was some cleaning up for me to do as he had messed in the hallway. He had also raised his leg in three or four other places. He was not on my treatment schedule this day, for the dog was only a boarder at the hospital that week. Just as I began to shuffle through the medical record cards of the cases that needed to be treated, the phone rang. Marna said that I had an accident case at this hospital and wanted to be certain that I had arrived. I asked her to call the service and have them instruct the party to come right down.

The hospital was cleaned up, and all the cases were treated when the Dahlborgs arrived with Kato, their Irish setter. They were directed to the nearest exam room, and Kato was placed on the table. Kato looked as if he might have rolled the length of a football field—he was covered with grass, leaves, and even some road oil. His front leg was askew and pointed as if he was planning to make a left turn. Exactly how bad the fracture was could only be determined by taking a radiograph. While the x-rays were being developed, I returned to the exam room and asked the Dahlborgs to assist me in completing the medical records.

The Dahlborgs had seen the accident. Kato had bounded across the street, and he was hit by a pick-up while in the middle of one of his "bounds." The wheel had hit his rear quarters, spun him around like a top, threw him against the curb and then against a tree. They emphatically told me that he was not run over—only hit by a car and thrown against hard objects.

The timer clock sounded in the darkroom, and I returned and brought the wet film out and checked it with the Dahlborgs on the viewing screen. The Dahlborgs were standing beside me as I looked at the film for the first time. Mr. Dahlborg took one look at the x-ray film, and returned to the reception room. His wife asked what all of those tiny "specks" were doing all over the film. I asked her if this was a hunting dog as the specks looked like buckshot to me. She said that Kato was at one time, but he had become frightened at the sound of gunfire, and had retired from hunting. Now he was just a household pet.

Mr. Dahlborg had been listening. He spoke up and said that he had accidentally shot Kato. That mistake had ruined him as a hunting dog.

Kato would not even get into the truck with him if he could smell gunpowder or recognize a gun.

A traction splint was fashioned to fit Kato's leg, and he was put into a cage for surgery tomorrow morning. While I had been preparing the splint, the owners had picked the grass and leaves from his coat. They gave him some loving pats as they prepared to say good-bye.

It was almost noon by the time I was ready to leave, and the clouds that had been in the northwest were now overhead. A light rain was beginning to fall. I knew that the boys would be disappointed about not having the picnic that Marna had promised.

As I entered the house, the boys came running, and said that we were going to have a picnic. I gave a quizzical glance at Marna and she responded with a nod. Now I really was puzzled!

My jacket was still over my arm, and I went to the hall closet to hang it up. There in the middle of the family room was a blanket on the floor. All of the chairs were pulled back to make room for it. A cooler chest and a picnic basket were on one corner of the blanket. Albert said, "Sit down Daddy." I sat down on one of the chairs. Immediately I was rebuffed by Allen who informed me that the chairs were really not there. Marna clarified the situation by saying that the boys were so disappointed in not going out for a picnic that they all agreed to have one at home. In essence, I could not see the chairs, the lamps, the walls, or the pictures that were hanging on them. Only green grass was "visible." The lamps had become trees and the chairs were gigantic boulders.

By this time the boys were sitting Indian fashion in their selected spots on the blanket. Marna was on her knees taking orders for peanut butter or tuna sandwiches. I joined them on the blanket. It was a great picnic. Coffee and soft drinks were available to go along with celery stalks, olives, and several kinds of chips. All of this was topped off with chocolate chip cookies that Marna had baked that morning.

It was great to be on this "in-house" picnic. George did spill his drink and Greta did get into the chips, but these were only minor inconveniences. My responsibility was to control the ants, and I must have done a superb job for none of us saw any.

We all helped with the cleanup. Folding the blanket was my chore. George and Albert carried the remaining food and utensils to the kitchen.

Allen was asked to let Greta outside for a run.

The sky was darker now and the rain began falling harder. Greta did not want to go out and no matter how much coaxing she received from Allen, she was determined to remain in the house. So we let Greta stay inside.

We didn't have a campfire during the picnic, but now that the weather was turning worse, I thought a fire in the fireplace would be cozy. We all sat down by the fire, but the boys did not remain there long. They had too much exuberance to remain still. Marna and I pulled a couple of chairs near the fire and Greta curled up in front of us. We had our extra cups of coffee and shared the morning's events. Soon we were out of conversation. Marna's head began to nod. My eyes were about to close—then the phone rang.

On the other end was a lady who owned one of these flop-eared rabbits—she said a cat had mangled it. Her conversation with me was delayed intermittently with bouts of crying. She was afraid that her bunny would have to be put to sleep. She wanted to meet me at the hospital for my opinion concerning her bunny's future.

San Pedro was about twenty minutes away, so I put on my rain gear and headed south. When I pulled into the hospital parking lot, she was already there. I went into the hospital and turned on the lights. The client did not come in. I went to the front door and could see her still sitting in her car. I put on my rain jacket and went out to assist her. She was sitting behind the wheel crying. A gray bundle of fur was lying motionless on her lap. I picked up the bunny and asked her to follow me. I could not feel a heartbeat and couldn't hear one with the stethoscope.

"What am I going to do now?" she asked. I explained to her that the hospital could take care of all the arrangements. She sat down and tried to compose herself. She said, "I was 'rabbit sitting' for my daughter. The rabbit was in the house all of the time, so I put it out in the fenced backyard in order that it might get some exercise. I felt it would be safe there. I heard this terrible squeal. I did not realize that rabbits make any noises, but I went out to investigate. A cat had it in its mouth and was getting ready to jump over the fence. I ran toward the cat. It released the rabbit and then scampered over the fence." She started crying again. I asked her if she would be able to drive home. She said, "Yes." Her greatest concern was informing her daughter what had happened. She left the hospital.

Even though I attempted to comfort her in her time of distress, I felt that I did a less than adequate job.

Later that night, I was connected to a dentist who had just been in an automobile accident. None of the human passengers had been hurt as they had been wearing seat belts. Another passenger, their show dog, a collie named Ranger, was unfortunately injured.

Ranger had three front teeth knocked out. He could not enter a show ring being disfigured in that manner unless corrections were made. The dentist needed some professional help. I was uncertain what his needs were. I listened carefully while he formulated a plan. If I could meet him at his dental clinic in an hour he would perform root canals. He heard that I had a portable gas anesthetic machine and he desired that I act as an anesthesioligist.

When I arrived at the dental office, the dentist was inside and Ranger was still in his car. The dentist went out to the car and retrieved Ranger. I had stopped at a hospital and borrowed a bottle of surital. This short-acting anesthetic was given intravenously and Ranger was connected to the metafane gas anesthetic machine machine that I carried with me in the customized trunk of my Mustang. The dentist proceeded with the root canals. Soon he had completed his work. We agreed that it would be best to stabilize the teeth with a plastic coating. I disconnected Ranger from the machine and placed him on the floor to recover.

We stepped across the street and visited over a cup of coffee while the dog was completing his recovery. Ranger had won numerous ribbons. His owner said that if nothing had been done to correct Ranger's teeth, he could liken the situation to a beauty contest where a beautiful blond was about to be crowned queen only to be disqualified when she smiled.

We returned to the hospital. Ranger was awake enough to be transported home, so I helped the dentist carry him out to his car. I recommended that Ranger stay on soft food for awhile and not be allowed to chew on anything. He agreed with me.

He asked me how he could compensate me. I said he owed me nothing. I had learned a great deal by observing and knew that I had gained a new friend. He said, "In that case, you are entitled to two courtesy dental hygienes at my office."

Watching a root canal surgery and participating only as an anesthesiologist were both new events for me. The dentist and I became good friends and I later sponsored his membership into the local Rotary Club.

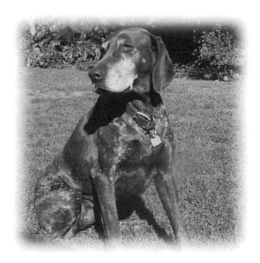

—26—

A No-Show

Marna always told me, "It is not what happens to you in life, but how you react to what happens to you that is important." This was excellent advice, but many times I failed to put it to use.

Clients would occasionally aggravate me. This evening was one of those nights. A gentleman was put through by the answering service. Immediately he started the conversation concerning the emergency call fee that the answering service had mentioned.

"It's a rip-off! You guys charge too much to begin with. Then to make matters worse, you add an emergency fee!" he said.

He continued, "Do you think I own a gold mine?"

I listened patiently until he had calmed down and then explained to him that the day charges were the same as night fees with the exception that an emergency fee was added in the off-hours of the hospital. This was to cover the cost that the doctor had incurred driving to and from the hospital.

"You mean that you don't live at the hospital?" he asked.

"No," I responded, "I live at home with my family."

"Well, okay, I can meet you at the Hawthorne hospital in about twenty minutes."

I agreed.

As I was driving to the hospital, I remembered that I had neglected to ask him the nature of the emergency.

When I arrived at Hawthorne, the phone was ringing. The operator informed me that the party had phoned back and cancelled the call. I got the party's number from the operator and contacted him directly.

He had indeed cancelled the call because he objected to the emergency fee. He did ask me that since I was already at the hospital, if he came down, would there still be an emergency fee? My response was a resounding, "Yes!" He hung up.

I never knew the nature of his reason for calling, and I was just as happy not having to confront him in person because of his attitude. I was smiling on the outside, and troubled on the inside as I arrived home an hour and a half later.

That evening, I had a return call to Hawthorne and George asked to ride with me. The Westfalls were coming in with their hunting dog, Bullet. Mr. Westfall had been hunting pheasants. Bullet had flushed one, and he had dropped it. When Bullet returned with the pheasant, he was limping on his right rear leg. Mr. Westfall thought that Bullet had only dinged his leg so he had resumed hunting. His dog continued to favor the leg. Bullet would walk on it gingerly, but when he tried to run on it, he limped noticeably.

I placed Bullet on the exam table and examined the leg. There was little pain involved, and he did not object when the leg was manipulated. Too much movement was discovered in the stifle (knee). I informed the owner that I was suspicious of a ruptured anterior cruciate ligament. (This ligament is frequently ruptured by athletes when it is exposed to excess stress.) A radiograph was taken, and my diagnosis was confirmed. Bullet was assigned to a cage. Surgery would take place the following day. I asked Mr. Westfall to call in the morning and inquire when surgery was to be scheduled.

George and I had to attend to another emergency in San Pedro before we headed home. A cat had a garage door close on it and now it could not walk. The Koroskys brought their cat into the hospital in a box. The cat was alert, but could not, or rather would not get up on its rear legs.

Carefully, I examined the cat to be certain that it had feeling in its rear quarters. If there was no sensation, there was a possibility of spinal injury. As I lifted a rear leg and rotated it slightly, Monty turned and severely bit my index finger on my right hand. There was excellent innervation to not only Monty's leg, but also to my finger. When rotating the leg, I had perceived some crepitation that indicated a fracture had occurred. I needed to take an x-ray to determine which bones had been broken.

I discussed the case with the Koroskys and we agreed that it would be best to keep Monty in the hospital and take x-rays in the morning. By doing it this way, Monty would have to have only one anesthetic. There was no way I could position him without sedation, and I knew that he had either a fractured leg or a fractured pelvis—or both. In the morning he would be sedated, x-rays would be taken, and he would immediately go in for surgical correction.

I gave Monty a tranquilizer injection of ketamine and acepromazine. George carried Monty and his box into the ward and placed them in a cage. The Koroskys were to call in the morning for an update.

My finger was now throbbing, so I soaked it in hot water and took a couple of ampicillin capsules to prevent infection. My finger felt somewhat better, but by the time I got home, it was throbbing again. The hot water soak was repeated. Monty's teeth had gone through the fingernail on one side and deep into the flesh on the other. For a week to ten days, my injured hand would render me useless as a surgeon, for I would not be able to hold any instruments with the proper dexterity.

Marna asked George what Daddy said when he was bitten. George replied, "Daddy said nothing. All he did was shake his hand and stare at the cat!"

Both George and I wondered where Allen and Albert were. Marna informed us that they were in the backyard bathing Greta. When I reached the backyard to greet the boys, the smell of skunk was evident. Both boys were in their swimsuits washing Greta. Allen had taken Greta for a walk, and they had confronted a skunk. I complimented them on the job they were doing, and rushed back to the house. Marna did not offer assistance either. We both watched the two boys from the porch while we consumed coffee.

George had decided to remain in the yard and give advice to his brothers. Before long, George let out a yell. Marna and I witnessed it all. Allen had squelched George with a bucket of soapy water. George then proceeded to grab the hose and squirt his brothers. Marna and I remained inside! Greta was forgotten as the boys concentrated on getting each other soaked. We remained on the safe side of the sliding door. We elected not to interfere, but after a period of time we called a halt to the frenzy and handed the boys some extra towels. They gave Greta a final rinse, toweled her down, and came into the house to take hot showers and settle down for the night.

The phone rang and the operator connected me with the Andrews. They owned a white cat named Silver whose ears were being bothered by flies. The flies had bitten her ears so badly that they were crusted around the edges and bleeding. To keep the flies away, she would shake her head. This action caused blood to be showered around the house. The Andrews said, "We put her outside to save the house. More flies were there and the problem increased. Now we are between a rock and a hard place and need your help." We agreed to meet at the hospital.

Silver and her owners were admitted. A beautiful Persian cat with big blue eyes was placed on the exam table. She had badly discolored ears and the hair around her ears was stained with blood. When I touched her ears, she immediately shook her head. Blood was sprayed over the adjacent wall. The next time I attempted to check her ears, I placed a towel over her head and carefully exposed one ear at a time for examination.

It did not appear to me that the flies were the initial problem. However, they were certainly adding to the aggravation. The ears of white cats are prone to skin cancer, and I felt that this was the proper diagnosis. Flies were attracted by the moisture of the cancerous lesions. Flies then make matters worse by biting the ears in the same area as the cancer.

The Andrews could not take care of their cat at home as she was destroying the house. Silver was left at the hospital for the night. The resident veterinarian would evaluate the case in the morning. Silver could shake her head all she wanted to and the mess could be easily cleaned off of the stainless steel cage—much easier than the furniture or carpet of a home. Also the hospital premises were fly-free so the two concerns would be under control.

27

SUPERCAT

The service had just connected me to the owners of Supercat. Supercat had just jumped through a window to catch a bird and had cut himself badly. It sounded like a "now" emergency, so I dropped what I was doing and headed for Manhattan Beach.

About half an hour after my arrival, the clients still had not arrived so I obtained their phone number from the service. I called them directly. There was no answer, so I could only assume that they were on their way. As I hung up the phone, they were pulling into the parking lot.

Both Mr. and Mrs. France came. Mr. France carried in a large aluminum cat carrier—the type used for airline transport. It appeared very heavy and he struggled with his load. I directed him to put the carrier on the exam table while I was getting information for the medical record from his wife. Supercat was his name. His breed was ocelot. I looked up and said, "Ocelot!" She said, "Yes!" An ocelot is a wild cat, native to South America and infrequently domesticated. His weight was forty-three pounds, and he was two and a half years old. With all of this information recorded, I realized that Supercat was really a supercat.

Mr. France was asked to get him out of the cage. He was unsuccessful. Mrs. France declined to try. Supercat was crouched in the back of his cage showing his teeth. I was hesitant about reaching into the cage when the Frances informed me that he had been declawed on all four feet. That helped to comfort me, but the ocelot still had to be removed from the cage in order for me to treat him. Four weapons had been nullified, but one remained—his teeth. I was gazing into the cage, and as he was "smiling" at me showing his pretty white teeth, he let out a deep-throated growl.

Elbow-length welding gloves were obtained from the treatment room. (This type of glove was kept on hand to protect our hands and arms from being scratched or bitten by the domestic cat.) These gloves might not protect me from his teeth to any great degree, but they gave me confidence.

By this time, Supercat was frightened and very defensive. The owners sweet-talked him by calling him "nice kitty" and the like. No headway was accomplished. He continued to seek refuge in the rear of his cage. Several fresh blood spots were now evident and it became apparent that he needed medical attention—that absolved my thought of declining to treat him.

Several times I reached in to grasp him by the neck and each time he would bat my gloved hand away with his paw like a boxer. I was amazed at the strength he had. Finally, I became aggressive enough to reach over him and drag him to the front of the cage by placing my gloved hand on his rump and pulling. I was unable to grasp him by the nape of the neck because of my gloves, but he did allow my hand to remain in that position. Mrs. France retrieved a blanket for me from the back of the hospital and Mr. France opened it up wide in front of himself. Now, as a team, we were ready. The next step was to pull Supercat the rest of the way out of the cage. When his head cleared the door of the cage, he leaped to the counter. Mr. France acted quickly and smothered him with the blanket. I had a syringe full of sedative ready, and now I administered the mixture of ketamine and acepromazine directly through the blanket into the muscle on the ocelot's rear leg. After almost twenty minutes, I was in complete control!

Up to that time, I never realized that my shirt was wet with perspiration from all the stress. Supercat had a deep cut on his chest and another cut on his back leg that needed suturing. Fur was trimmed away, and I worked in a hurried fashion to perform the necessary surgery. I did not wish to give a general anesthetic as ocelots and other wild animals occasionally do not respond to them in the prescribed manner.

I placed a terry cloth towel on the floor of his cage, and then put the ocelot gently on it. By this time, Supercat was looking at me with a blank stare and flexing his paws. My timing had been perfect, for he was rapidly waking up.

The Frances said they would leave the cage door open when they arrived home, so Supercat could come out whenever he was mobile. He would be in his own surroundings, and he would not be reluctant to venture out.

An appointment was made for suture removal in two weeks. A red star was placed by Supercat's name to warn the staff that the ocelot could be dangerous to handle. I mentioned to the Frances that I wished I had brought a camera, for the boys would have been interested in seeing a picture of an ocelot. They told me thay had many pictures of Supercat at their home and they would be happy to mail some to me. I gave them my home address.

Marna was surprised when I told her about the case. The boys were more than excited. I located a cardboard box and a pair of garden gloves. I acted out the entire affair. The boys sat around and were very attentive. My acting took nearly thirty minutes. I used a stuffed cat to represent the ocelot. When "surgery" was done and I put the stuffed animal back into the cage and locked the door, I said "amen." Albert quickly said, "Do it again, Daddy!" Marna laughed and diverted their attention with a serving of graham crackers and hot chocolate.

We were still laughing and drinking hot chocolate when the phone rang. Mr. Lopez called and asked me to see his dog, Diablo (which means devil). He thought Diablo had something stuck in his mouth or throat. I asked if he would look into his dog's throat and see if anything was visible. "Diablo won't let me," was his response. We agreed to meet at the Gardena hospital in thirty minutes.

The clients arrived first. They were walking Diablo around the parking lot on a leash. Diablo was about a ninety-pound black pit bull. As I walked by him on the way to unlock the front door, he welcomed me with a low-pitched warning growl.

I decided to give him a wide berth as we entered the hospital. He immediately went over to the nearest chair and raised his leg. The owner jerked the leash, and Diablo turned toward me and growled again.

When the paperwork was completed, we proceeded to the examination room. Dog and master were allowed to enter first, for I had no intention of being trapped without an avenue of escape. I asked Mr. Lopez to lift Diablo's front end, which contained the teeth and the growl, and I volunteered to pick up the rear portion of his dog. Mr. Lopez asked me to stand out of the way while he put his dog on the table by himself. I appreciated his thoughtfulness.

There was no way I would be able to examine Diablo's mouth area unless he was fast asleep. The owner agreed wholeheartedly with my decision to sedate his dog. Mrs. Lopez had remained in the reception room while her husband handled their dog. Diablo's head was turned toward the wall, and with Mr. Lopez holding him securely, I slipped up on the dog's near side using Mr. Lopez's body as a shield and injected a sedative intramuscularly in Diablo's rear leg.

Ever so slowly, Diablo began to melt into Mr. Lopez's arms, and silently he began to relax until he was now in a prone position on the exam table. My intention was to examine his mouth immediately and if nothing was noted then to give a general anesthetic and check his throat. To our mutual relief, a bone was located in his mouth. The bone had lodged securely between his upper teeth like a bridge from one side of his mouth to the other. It was fixed so tightly against his hard palate that it could not be removed manually. I located a piece of oak doweling and gently leveraged it out from between his teeth.

During this foreign body removal process, Mr. Lopez had been talking to his wife in Spanish. As soon as the bone was removed, he asked me what the charges were. He related that information to his wife in Spanish, and she wrote a check. He was in a hurry because he wanted to get Diablo home before he woke up. "Diablo is unpredictable and sometimes is very mean," was his comment.

Now I was able to help lift Diablo. Mr. Lopez and I carried him out to the pick-up. Mrs. Lopez handed me the check and they were off.

Earlier Mr. Lopez related to me that Diablo had been trained to not be friendly. This was apparent and greatly troubled me. Mrs. Lopez only weighed slightly more than their dog and there was no way she could restrain him. Diabalo would not even respond to her commands. If Diablo ever got out of his premises, there was no way she could pull him off a person or more specifically a child. Many times during a year, the newspapers carry stories about a dog or dogs attacking children. Diablo was big and strong enough to do considerable damage to anyone. This black pit bull was potentially a menace to the community.

—28—

UNDER
SURVEILLANCE

It had been a long day at the hospital. My surgery was completed after hours. I grabbed my coat and was locking up when the phone rang. The operator connected me to a client from the Hermosa Beach hospital. She wanted me to examine her puppy, which had crawled under her couch and chewed on an electrical extension cord.

Instead of heading for home, I headed in the opposite direction to Hermosa. The cocker spaniel pup was more frightened than hurt. Mild electrical burns were on his face and tongue. I rubbed in some soothing furacin ointment into the facial lesions and dispensed some of the same. Since the lesion was hard to treat in his mouth and the mouth usually heals well, I suggested that soft food be fed for a few days.

The owner told me that she heard the puppy cry out and didn't think much of it until she entered her living room. At this point, she noticed the floor lamp by the couch had a light flickering. She decided to change the bulb. When she returned with the new bulb, there was a burning smell in the room. Wisely she unplugged the light and checked its extension cord under the couch. The pup had chewed on the cord, and there were scorched marks on the carpet. Fortunately she was at home and averted the possibility of a house fire.

With this case behind me, I headed for home. It was dark when I arrived at my destination. Marna met me at the door saying that the service was still on the line and would wait a moment for me to get to the phone.

A woman was calling from a pay phone near the Torrance hospital about a dog she may have killed. The operator cross-connected me and all I could make out was, "I've killed Teddy! I've killed him! Please come right away." As I hung up, Marna handed me a "sack dinner" which she had hurriedly prepared. I immediately embarked for that hospital.

When I arrived, Mrs. Gault was sitting on the front planter box with a Chihuahua cradled on her lap. I unlocked the door and indicated for her to follow me. She did not respond. She just sat there with the dog on her lap, rocking back and forth exclaiming, "I've killed him! I've killed him!" I grabbed the dog from her arms and headed for the treatment room. I invited her to follow.

Once in the treatment room, I rolled the oxygen tank over, entubated the dog, and began positive resuscitation. In the meantime, Mrs. Gault had followed me in and was leaning against the wall crying. No response was elicited. Next I gave an injection of epinepherine intracardially to stimulate a heartbeat. No response. I decided to give another injection into the heart. I turned around to get the vial again and bumped headlong into an officer of the law. He quickly got out of my way. I gave the second injection. Still no response. Teddy had died.

While I had been treating the Chihuahua, a police officer had been standing there watching me. He and two other cars had responded to an alarm that had been relayed to them. An apartment owner nearby had called the police about a lady who was standing in front of the hospital saying that she had killed Teddy. The officers were investigating. They asked Mrs. Gault and me to remain where we were and then he asked my permission to look around the facility.

While the officers were inspecting the premises, Mrs. Gault had become more lucid. Mrs. Gault was a self-appointed veterinarian. Somewhere she had procured a vial of penicillin. Her dog was sick and she gave him an injection. Her three-pound dog should only have been administered a half milliliter of the antibiotic, but she had given three milliliters of penicillin to her tiny dog. She felt that if a little antibiotic did a good job, then a lot of antibiotic would do a better job. (I suspected that some had accidentally been injected intravenously which will cause an immediate fatality.) She was also handicapped in her judgment—she had consumed too much John Barleycorn. To be more exact, she was also a bit inebriated. She did request that I release the dog to her in order that she might bury him at home. She took Teddy in her arms and headed for her car.

The officers, five in all, were still at the hospital. They were looking at each other. I was certain that she would be given a ticket for driving under the influence as soon as she pulled out of the driveway onto a public street. Before she started her car, I suggested that she let me drive her home in my car. Mrs. Gault would not leave her car at the hospital overnight.

The officer that I had bumped into in the hospital came to my aid. He offered to follow in his patrol car as I drove her home and then bring me back to the hospital to retrieve my Mustang.

Soon I was on my way home with my "sack dinner" still by my side. Marna sat down with me at the kitchen table while I ate my supper and related the night's experience to her.

Before long, I had another emergency call. The service connected me with the Gleasons. Boots, their cat, could not seem to keep her food down. "She eats, and about an hour later, she 'pukes' it up," was their graphic explanation. Boots also seemed to be getting weaker. She was lying around the house more than usual. This also worried them, for Boots was usually a very active cat.

We agreed to meet at the Torrance hospital in thirty minutes. When they arrived, I filled out the medical report and we traversed as a team into the exam room. Boots was indeed sick. "She may have this flu that has been going around," said Mrs. Gleason as she attempted to assist me in the diagnosis.

Boots was very dehydrated, and she did not object when I palpated her abdomen. There was a suspicious bulge in her intestinal tract that I could not identify. I relayed to the Gleasons that there appeared to be a foreign body of some unknown origin located in her intestine. It would be appropriate to take an x-ray of her gastrointestinal system using barium as a contrast medium. They were not sure they wanted to make that kind of investment, but after we discussed the symptoms and my observations, they approved when I told them that an intestinal blockage was usually fatal.

A powdered barium sulfate was mixed with water into a thick solution. A stomach tube was passed enabling all of the medium to be deposited directly into the stomach. Six lateral x-ray views were taken at fifteen-minute intervals. I then evaluated the sequence of film.

The radio-opaque mixture could be seen in the stomach and in the anterior part of the small intestine. At one location, the solution did not pass down the tract any further. The last three views were almost identical. There was an obvious blockage caused by some soft object, for it was not dense enough to suggest a ball or a rock. The Gleasons tried to figure out what the object could be.

Suddenly the Gleasons came up with a possible solution. Mrs. Gleason had to keep her hose picked up, for Boots liked to chew them up. "Could it possibly be something of this nature?" Mrs. Gleason asked. This question supported my provisional diagnosis even more. I told the Gleasons that at this stage, I could not confirm exactly what the blockage was caused by, but a blockage was definitely evident.

I recommended surgery and the Gleasons reluctantly agreed with me that there was no other way to relieve Boots of her problem. An intravenous drip of a saline solution was connected to relieve her dehydration and also supply some potassium to her system. Surgery was prepared for an enterotomy.

I showed Mrs. Gleason where the coffee maker was and invited her to make coffee for herself and her husband.

An hour later, Boots was sporting a sutured ventral midline incision and I was removing my surgical gloves. The intravenous drip was still connected. I changed the solution from saline to five-percent dextrose and saline. I carried Boots into the recovery room, rolling the intravenous drip stand with me as I did so. I placed her in the cage with her right foot extended so that the connecting tubing of the drip system would not get tangled.

Before talking to the Gleasons, I rinsed off the piece of ladies' hose that I had recovered and was able to identify. Then I poured a cup of coffee and went to the front of the hospital. They were dumbfounded that Boots would ingest something like that. Holes had been chewed in Mrs. Gleason's hose before, but they had not noticed any pieces missing.

We walked back to the ward and found Boots resting comfortably. She was beginning to wake up—I could elicit an eyelid reflex. The intravenous feeding would remain during the night, but I reduced the flow to one drop every five seconds. The Gleasons were to call the office in the morning for a progress report. Boots would be on a soft diet for several days. The doctor who discharged their cat would go over her aftercare in detail.

We mutually agreed that Boots would not relate her surgery to her chewing habit. Therefore it would be necessary to be extra careful in keeping hose out of her reach. "Why were you so certain that she had swallowed cloth or nylon?" asked the Gleasons. My response was "experience," for this was the fourth time I had done surgery for this kind of problem. For some unknown reason, cats have an affinity for chewing on hose. My previous surgeries had all been performed on Siamese cats. This was the first time that I had witnessed this problem on a different breed.

It had been a long night. Since I had heard the phone ring while I was in surgery, I called the answering service to let them know I was out of surgery and now available. The operator told me that it was an urgent emergency and that she had referred the owners to another hospital.

I rarely missed cases, but it was impossible to be at two places at the same time. Sometime in the future an emergency hospital would have to be established where a veterinarian would be in attendance at all times. In the years ahead, that dream may become a reality.

When I got home, Keith had been trying to reach me. He owned the hospital where I had treated the ocelot. He wanted to know how I had gotten that darn ocelot out of his cage. He had tried for over half an hour to get Supercat out of his cage so he could remove the sutures. He never got the cat out. The stitches had remained where I put them. The Frances had suggested that Supercat would not be so hyper at home and maybe they could remove the sutures themselves. Keith agreed with the owners, for the ocelot, in its own environment, would be much easier to handle. Keith said that he had requested the owners call him and describe the surgical sites so he could make proper entries on Supercat's medical record.

29

THE RED BALL

When leaving for an emergency, it was important to make haste. Occasionally there were delays such as changing a flat tire, running out of gas, and even waiting for a train. Sometimes I forgot the hospital keys. This time the delay was of a completely different nature. I was to meet the Robertses, who owned a rottweiler with a very fast growing tumor on the side of his face. I arrived at the hospital first and found a large German shepherd chained to the front door handle.

The only key that I had for that hospital was for that door. The shepherd was frightened and defensive. She would not let anyone near her. Soft talking made little difference. As soon as I would make a motion toward her, she would show her teeth and the hair at the back of her neck would stand on edge. I was certainly in a quandary as to what to do to gain entry to the hospital.

My client arrived with his rottweiler. I asked him to leave his dog in the car. Then we consulted. Since his case was not a life or death matter, we decided to work as a team to outfox the "sentry" dog. He brought over the leash from his dog and was able to loop it over the shepherd's neck. Next I located a large piece of cardboard in the trash and used it as a shield. Mr. Roberts pulled the shepherd with his leash to one side as I protected myself with the cardboard. I was then able to insert the key and open the door. I entered the hospital, locked the front door from the inside, went to the rear of the hospital, and opened the back door. My client with his rottweiler was now inside.

119

I immediately called the Humane Society and asked them to come over and get the abandoned shepherd. (There was no way that I would bring the shepherd into the hospital. Once it had gained entry, the hospital would have to take care of it for thirty days before it could be released to the Humane Society. As long as it remained outside, it was classified as an abandoned pet.)

We put the rottweiler up on the exam table to examine the swelling on the right side of his cheek. I checked his temperature and it was high. I then checked his mouth, and there was a purulent exudation from the edge of one of his molars. My diagnosis was an abscessed tooth.

The owner held his dog while I administered the intravenous sedative. The molar was extracted and the abscess lanced. A seton was placed to insure that drainage would continue. Ointment was put into the abscessed area and the antibiotic, ampicillin, was given in the muscle. As the lanced area was draining considerably, I suggested that the dog remain in the hospital overnight.

I was overruled. The owner informed me that the dog was very hard to handle when away from his owners. So he paid his bill and we then carried the seventy-pound-plus dog out the back door and placed him in the station wagon. I was glad the owner had informed me of the rottweiler's temperament—I would have felt awful if one of the morning attendants or the doctor had been bitten unexpectedly.

As I was returning to the hospital, the Humane Society officer arrived. He was experienced and released the shepherd from the front door in no time at all. The dog was put in the Humane Society's truck and carted off. I locked the back door and exited through the front door, locking it this time from the outside. I took a leisurely drive home down the coast.

The sun was just setting over the Pacific Ocean and the clouds made the sunset picture perfect. As I opened the back door, Marna asked if I had seen the sunset. All five of us went out into the yard and observed the sun as it disappeared from the sky. The sunset lasted a little longer. We all marveled at God's creation.

Just about the time the sunset disappeared from the western sky, the telephone rang. Another case was scheduled for me—in San Pedro. I got ready to leave and the phone rang again. I suspected that the client had cancelled the call as they had seemed rather hesitant after the emergency fee was quoted. Another call was on my agenda in Torrance so I scheduled the second one forty minutes after the first one. I was on my way south to the harbor. Neither case was very unusual. The first was a cat that had a bite wound from a cat fight, and the Torrance case was a dog with a foxtail in her left ear. I pulled back into the garage about ten o'clock and was able to spend the rest of the evening with the family.

Early the next morning, I was talking to the Jansens on the telephone. They said that their dog, Fredie, had something stuck in his mouth. When I got to the Torrance hospital, the Jansens were waiting in their car. Fredie was a black and tan doxie. Mrs. Jansen carried him into the hospital.

We stopped long enough at the front desk to record the necessary paperwork, and then proceeded to the exam room. I was shaking down the mercury in the thermometer when I saw a flash of red near Fredie's mouth. I looked carefully and saw nothing. Then when he opened his mouth again, I saw a red ball. The ball appeared to be attached to his tongue!

I examined Fredie's mouth more intently. The tongue was securely attached to a little red rubber ball about the size of a golf ball. The Jansens said that the ball was his "squeaker" toy. "He would bite the ball and it would emit a definite squeak. Fredie carried the ball all over the house. He seemed to enjoy sneaking up behind us and squeaking the ball. If we jumped when he did this, he appeared delighted. Sometimes he would just lay on the floor or in a chair and chew on the ball—the noise would drive us crazy. About a week ago, the ball lost its metal squeaker. We have never found it, but that did not stop Fredie, for he would still carry the ball around the house chewing on it in hopes that it would squeak again. Yesterday the ball disappeared. When we got home from work tonight, we noticed that he had not touched his food. We thought that he was sick and were consoling him when we noticed the ball stuck on his tongue."

I examined Fredie's mouth more closely. The tongue and ball were attached to each other too firmly to pull the ball loose. In squeezing the ball, a vacuum had been created and the tongue was sucked inside the ball. Fredie was sedated with surital and connected to the gas anesthetic machine. I relieved the negative pressure within the ball by taking a nick out of the ball with surgical scissors. I enlarged the "squeaker" hole slightly and slid the ball from the tongue. The tip of the tongue was now visible. The slate gray color of the tip of the tongue indicated that vascular circulation had been impeded. It was necessary to amputate nearly an inch of tongue back to where the tissue was viable. Even after excising the tip of tongue, it did not bleed. No sutures were needed and I allowed the tongue to heal on its own. I had never seen or heard of a case like this before—it was definitely a first for me.

I returned to the front of the hospital to discuss the aftercare with the Jansens. Soft food would be required for a few days. It would be hard for Fredie to pick up food and even more difficult for him to lap water. I suggested that they put his water pan at shoulder height so he could get a mouthful of water, and then hold his nose high letting the water run down his throat like a bird drinks. We discussed several other options that should be considered. The Jansens were to call the hospital in a few days and let them know about Fredie's progress in eating and drinking. I locked the hospital door as we left and then all of us headed for our homes.

I was at the Gardena hospital for my next case. It was almost impossible not to laugh when I saw my patient. It was not the abscess on its front paw that was amusing to me. What was humorous was the cat's appearance. It was a shorthaired gray cat that had a strip of gray fur down the center of its back with the grain of the hair flowing contrary to the rest of its fur. It looked like a feline Rhodesian Ridgeback. Someone might have given it a Mohawk haircut.

When the owners noted the expression on my face, they remarked that several years ago she had experienced a skin graft to replace some missing skin on her back. It was a swing graft so the skin containing the hair had been turned around, changing the direction of her coat. Now she had hair flowing in two directions.

Show-and-tell was now over and my curiosity was satisfied. It was now time to address the emergency problem. Mable's foot was about three times its normal size, and she was unable to walk on it. She was a very docile cat so we decided to wrap her in a towel and try to lance the abscess without administering a sedative. The foot was exposed, and the owners held the leg so it was stabilized and extended. In a matter of minutes, I lanced the foot and drained the abscess. A seton was established so the abscess could continue to drain. I applied forte ointment to the abscess and an antibiotic injection of penicillin was given in the muscle.

Mable was discharged. I recommended that she be kept in the garage or any other place where the wound would not be contaminated and where she would not track the discharge around creating a mess.

When I left the hospital I happened to drive by another hospital, and I noticed my colleague's car in the parking lot. I parked my car and rapped on the front door. Don had just completed an emergency and was cleaning up surgery. We chatted for awhile and then realized we were both hungry. We stopped at a nearby restaurant and enjoyed a sandwich and a cup of coffee as we continued our conversation. After we had brought each other up on our personal events, we departed and headed home.

About bedtime, I was on my way again. The McLains had a cocker spaniel that needed attention. They could not ascertain exactly what the problem was—every time they wanted to look at Ruff's foot, she would circle and sit down so it could not be observed. If they tried to be more forceful, she would growl at them. Since Ruff was being so protective of her foot, they knew something was really bothering her.

Ruff allowed us to pick her up and place her on the exam table. We could do anything to her, as long as it did not involve her left rear foot. A piece of gauze was used to tie her mouth. This safety procedure would protect both the owners and myself from any defensive action on her part.

Ruff had been licking her dewclaw and considerable saliva was present. The McLains held her carefully while I examined her sore foot. She had two dewclaws on that particular foot, and both of them had grown around in a circle and penetrated the flesh. The area was badly inflamed and had to be extremely painful.

An open-ended nail trimmer was used to clip the nails. The distal portion of the nail was extracted from the fleshy part of the foot. I applied the topical antibiotic, liquachlor, and wrapped the foot securely to control the bleeding. An antibiotic injection of ampicillin was given, and I was about to remove her mouth gag when I thought it would be a good idea to check the rest of her feet. The rest of her nails were trimmed. None of them were yet causing any problem. I removed the gauze from her mouth and she growled at me—obviously she was not thanking me for my effort! I recommended that Ruff's feet be checked on a regular basis. They could purchase nail trimmers at any pet shop, and I had already demonstrated how to secure Ruff's mouth with gauze in case she would not allow them to handle her feet. I instructed them to remove the bandage in two days, and then call the office and give them a report.

I phoned Marna to see if I had any more calls. She did not answer. I had remembered her saying earlier in the day that the pantry was almost bare and she had planned to go to the grocery store. She usually shopped at one store in particular, so I thought I would go there and surprise her. I recognized her car in the parking lot, so I left a note under the windshield wipers that asked her to meet me at the nearby yogurt shop. Soon she was coming in the door of the yogurt shop with a big smile on her face. I had ordered her favorite—low-fat vanilla with chocolate sauce—ahead of time and asked it to be served when my wife arrived.

We were only a block or so from the ocean so we decided to take our yogurts down to the beach, sit on a bench, and watch the sunset. We lost track of time and responsibility, for after monitoring the beautiful sunset, we continued to sit there together. Finally reality outweighed desire and we headed home. I stopped to pick up a pizza for the boys, while Marna went home to put the food away. She let our sons know that I would be home soon with a special treat.

After the pizza had been demolished, Allen decided to organize a game of Monopoly with his brothers. He counted all the money and divided it fairly. The houses and hotel sales were to be managed by Allen as he was the banker. A little wrangling took place before the game began. Allen made up the rules. Ten minutes later, he walked by with the Monopoly game in a box and said that George and Albert decided not to play. Marna and I laughed.

—30—

BATHING PUPPIES

Sunday was here again, and I was up early to take care of the treatments at several hospitals. In the summertime I was more involved with Sunday and holiday treatments. Other veterinarians had outings planned with their families or commitments of some other nature. I completed my rounds and returned home to take Marna and the boys to church at eleven. I dutifully notified the answering services where I could be reached and the ushers where I would be sitting. I was not called out on an emergency during the entire service. Marna and I decided it was a day of rest for me too, so instead of heading home, we took the boys to brunch.

It was a pleasant morning and it was great to spend some time with the boys. We ate at a little restaurant along the coast. The boys were excited about watching the waves break on the sandy beach. Fishermen were walking in the surf with scoop nets catching fish of some kind. It was interesting watching footprints appear in the sand as the joggers went by—then incoming waves would wash them away. George likened it to a slate—he would make an entry, then wipe it off with an eraser.

Brunch was a lively time as each of the boys seemed to have something to say—at the same time. Marna or I would continually have to call a halt to the confusion and say, "It is now George's time to talk" (then Albert's, or then Allen's). We had finished eating and Marna and I were enjoying another cup of coffee. Allen was giving his brothers instruction in coloring with the crayons that had been provided.

Our waitress brought me the bill. She asked if I was the doctor who was anticipating a phone call. (When we arrived at the restaurant, I had called and given the answering services the telephone number. I had also told the hostess that I might receive a telephone call.) The service was calling about a case at the nearby Palos Verdes hospital. The client's dog had something in its ear and was in discomfort. I took care of the account and went outside and assisted Marna in getting the boys into her car. I watched them leave and then got into my Mustang to make the journey to Palos Verdes.

Directly in front of my car was a woman driving with a child in a car seat beside her. On top of her car was her purse. I honked and pointed toward the top of her car. She glanced in her rearview mirror and preferred to ignore me. At the next signal, I was able to change lanes and pull up beside her car. I reached across and rolled down my window on the passenger side and tried to get her attention. I waved at her and pointed to the purse on top her car. She rolled up the window of her car and stared straight ahead. I honked once more, but she would not even glance in my direction.

A man had pulled up behind her and noted what I was trying to do. Before the signal could change, he got out of his car, walked up to the driver's side, and knocked on her window. She jumped with alarm! He was able to convey to her that her purse was still on top of her car. She recovered her purse, and finally looked in my direction. I could read her lips as she said, "Thank you," over the din of traffic. I was pleased with the results of my "good deed" and the assistance I received from the unknown driver. A smile was on my face as I pulled into the hospital's parking lot.

Most of the time when I arrived at hospital on an emergency, the owners were pleased to see me. Today my experience was different. Mrs. West seemed happy, but her husband was less than overjoyed.

Dee Dee had her head tilted to her left side, and this indicated to me that her left ear troubled her. Mrs. West did an exceptional job of holding Dee Dee and soon I was holding a foxtail that I had recovered. All this time, Mr. West stood leaning against the wall with his arms crossed.

As is my habit, I recommended that we look at the other ear as well. She turned Dee Dee around, and as I picked up the otoscope again, her husband said, "What are you trying to do—create more income?" I ignored his remark and continued my examination. Soon I had retrieved another foxtail. I showed it to Mrs. West, and I knew that her husband was taking all of this in. I didn't flaunt the foxtail in front of him, but I did look in his direction. He remained stationary in his original position supporting the wall and grunted.

Some panalog was put in each ear and the rest of the tube was sent home with Mrs. West. Something was troubling Mr. West. Finally, I was able to engage him in a conversation.

"Why do you charge fifteen dollars for an emergency?" he asked.

I now realized what was bothering him. I explained to him, as I had done to others, that it was my compensation for the extra time involved.

"That is not good business," was his next remark. He continued to bombard me with insinuations and other uncalled for remarks. I decided not to comment and remained silent. Mrs. West was taking all of this in, but did not venture into the discussion. Her husband kept it up and remained with his arms folded across his chest as he leaned against the wall. I was beginning to become irritated. Suddenly, I thought of a good approach—the best defense is a good offense. I started to distract him by asking questions.

"What do you do for a living?"

"I have my own television repair service."

"Where is it located?"

"In Hermosa Beach."

"Do you have to go out in off-hours?"

"On occasion."

"What's the extra charge for these trips?"

Before he could answer, his wife blurted out, "Twenty-two fifty."

He now understood the direction of my questions. He had never expected his wife to intervene in the conversation. A cold stare at his wife revealed his displeasure with her unsolicited response. I never heard him utter another word while he was in the hospital.

He paid for the services in cash. He didn't offer any sign of gratitude, but I didn't expect any either.

They left and I cleaned the premises.

I drove home thinking about the couple. Perhaps Mr. West was reprimanding his wife or perhaps it was a very quiet ride for both of them. In either case, I was amused at her intervening comment. Marna heard my story about the Wests over a cold glass of iced tea.

I took my iced tea outside and sat down in a lawn chair. I glanced over at my Mustang and noted that it was filthy. It needed a bath, and Allen offered to assist me. I was just washing the last of the suds from the car when I was greeted by Mr. Jansen. He was out walking Fredie on a leash. We talked about Fredie's progress.

He said that Fredie was eating solid food well. He would grab a mouthful and toss it into the air, catch it, chew it, and then swallow it. It took him a bit of time to eat, but he was managing. Consuming water was a different matter. He would not drink water by tipping his head back like a bird and letting it run down his throat, as I had suggested. "I made a special device for him—sort of a drinking fountain." Mr. Jensen tried to explain the apparatus to me, but I could not envision what he was describing.

Mr. Jansen lived only two blocks away, and he invited me to come to his house and inspect his handiwork. Allen volunteered to rinse the car off and towel it down. We walked to his house.

Mr. Jansen asked me to call him "Bob." Bob was a retired engineer and very creative. He had run some copper tubing from an outside waterline (in the same manner that an icemaker is installed in a refrigerator). He had affixed a pedal to regulate the water flow. Fredie could now drink water whenever he wanted and no water would be wasted. All he had to do was step on the pedal of his newly designed canine drinking fountain. The end of the tube was head-high, enabling water to almost trickle down his throat. He only had to instruct Fredie two or three times before his dog mastered the procedure.

We enjoyed a good cold beer and visited for over an hour. Bob had worked as an engineer for Boeing for thirty-five years and had been retired for twelve. When I returned home, Marna was upset. I had just disappeared without letting her know where I was going. I vowed it would not happen again and I apologized for my sojourn down the street to Bob's house.

Several times in the years ahead, I saw or spoke to Bob Jansen. One day he was walking without Fredie. I was heading in the opposite direction and waved to him as I passed. He was walking slowly using a cane. He waved back. That was the last time I saw him. Whenever I washed the car, I frequently thought of Bob, Fredie, and the red ball.

Later that afternoon, I was spending time with the boys and Marna. Frequently I received calls from the various answering services, but it was not always necessary to respond to a call in person. I had two phone conversations with clients that afternoon. After the second, I returned to the backyard to continue playing catch with the football with Allen. The fall season had just started and the television set became a very important fixture for the men of the family. Interest seemed to rest on the subject of football. Football was in the air as well as on the air. In the backyard, Allen was the quarterback—I was the center. The younger two were wide receivers. Allen said that his receivers were "not much good" for they rarely caught the ball. Allen was not very accurate, so his completion percentage was very low.

Marna came to the yard and called a time-out in order for me to get to the phone. While I talked, the rest of the team suggested that Mother should be the "water girl" and that some Gatorade needed to be brought out to the players.

The Jacksons were on the phone—they had a dog named Blossom that had a litter of pups. The pups were not doing well. One pup had died this morning and the rest were very weak. Two were so weak they could not nurse. George and Albert wanted to go with me to see the puppies. Allen had something else he wanted to do, so the three of us headed west to the Redondo Beach hospital.

Blossom's seven pups were brought into the hospital in a box. I had inferred that Blossom should accompany them, but apparently did not make that request clear enough. The box full of pups was placed on the exam table.

I picked up the first pup and noted that it was covered with fleas. The pup was very anemic as its mucous membranes were almost completely white—not a normal rosy pink. Fleas were bleeding the pups to death. I had George start bathing the first pup. I sent the Jacksons home with some flea shampoo to bathe Blossom and some yard spray to use on the bedding and premises. Between the boys and me, we bathed all the pups. I put mineral oil in each of the pup's eyes to keep them from being irritated by the shampoo. George did the bathing. He applied the shampoo and lathered each pup one at a time. Albert took each pup to a cage so it could soak—allowing all the fleas to be killed. When this was done to the entire litter, Albert brought each pup back out in the original order and George rinsed the pup off and handed it to me for drying. We became very efficient by the time we had completed this process on all seven. All the fleas had been removed and the pups were dry by the time the Jacksons returned. We put their cardboard box in the trash and located a new one and lined it with a clean towel.

Albert put the wet towels in the washing machine and George cleaned up the room. I sent George down to the corner to buy some refreshments to quench our thirsts. The Jacksons said that they thought the flea problem at home was under control. They had noted a lot of "red, wine-colored" water when they washed Blossum. I explained that the dried blood from the flea's stools had been dissolved in the water.

The pups were now dry and ready to go home. Before they were discharged, I gave each of them a feeding of five-percent glucose subcutaneously. I sent some liquid vitamins home for supportive care.

"Why did you let this flea problem continue for such a long time?" I asked. Mrs. Jackson said that Blossom had her pups in a secluded corner of the garage and that they did not want to interfere with her care of them. She added, "I thought that Mother Nature could adequately take care of the nursing mother and her pups. When Blossom came out to eat this morning, I peeked in to see how many pups she had. There was one dead pup and these seven weak ones. My husband called you because the rest looked sick, and we did not wish to lose any more. We felt that we should not rely any longer on 'the survival of the fittest.'"

I told them that when they got home to hold each pup in the nursing position until they were strong enough to do so themselves. "Be sure that Blossom has an adequate supply of milk for the pups. In fact, call me about nine this evening and let me know what kind of progress you have made. If the pups need a supplement, I will recommend one to you then." (They did call me later that night and told me that two more had died. Later I was informed that the remaining five had reached the age of six weeks.)

George and Albert immediately bragged to Allen about the pups when we got home. George had bathed seven and Albert had dried nine. It took a few minutes to convince Albert that there were only seven pups so he could not have dried more than that. As the boys were leaving the family room, Albert told Allen, "I really dried nine pups!"

—31—

A "Dog Doctor"

On this blustery night, I was heading north in my Mustang. I was not too mindful of my speed or what was happening around me. It was almost midnight and the roads were free of traffic, and I was in a hurry to reach my destination.

I didn't know too much about the case. The owners had been rather excitable so I did not quiz them to the normal degree. I was mulling over in my mind about the problem their cocker spaniel had and trying to piece together the information I was able to glean from my conversation with the client. My brain just couldn't get in gear and come up with a plausible analysis.

I wasn't paying much attention until an intermittent red light illuminated the interior of the car. I put on the right-turn signal and eased my Mustang over to the right searching for an open place along the curb. The officer approached my side of the car and asked to see my driver's license.

I obtained the document he had requested from my wallet and handed it to him. The officer broke the silence by asking me if I knew why he had pulled me over. I replied that I must have been going too fast.

"Why are you in such a hurry?" he asked.

"I am on my way to the hospital to treat an emergency case that is already in transit," I answered.

"Do you have something to indicate you are a doctor?" was his next question.

I showed him my membership card for the local veterinary chapter. He looked at the card carefully and remarked, "Well, what do you know, a dog doctor!"

He indicated to me that I could be on my way, and warned me about driving too fast. I thanked him and pulled away from the curb continuing my way to the Hawthorne hospital.

Just as I was unlocking the hospital door, lights from the client's car played across the front of the building. I had arrived in time, despite my delay.

The owner and my patient were taken immediately into the exam room. The Smyths had let Moocher out of their trailer at the trailer park so he could do his evening chore. Their favorite television program was on, so they had returned to watch it. As they were sitting there engrossed in the program, the screen dimmed, got brighter, and then dimmed again. It was possible that the entire park was experiencing electrical difficulties, so they opened their door to see if others were having a similar problem. They stepped out on the ground, then noticed Moocher with the electrical tie-line in his mouth. His wife screamed and went over to pull Moocher out from under the trailer. A neighbor restrained her and told her not to touch the dog. He then went around the trailer and disconnected the electrical power.

"Moocher had been rigid with all four feet extended, and he was quivering. When the power was turned off, he relaxed. I took him into the trailer thinking he had been electrocuted. I thought he was a dead, but his eyes were open and he was blinking them. He could not walk or otherwise move. We then called you."

Moocher had a gray burn lesion on each side of his face and there was an inch-wide brand across the top of his tongue. His heart rate was slow and his breathing shallow. He was beginning to move slightly. It appeared that he was aware of what was happening to him now. He was making a feeble effort to get upright on his chest. Their neighbor had saved Moocher from being electrocuted and quite likely saved Mrs. Smyth from the same fate.

I treated Moocher for the obvious lesions and sent home some salve to rub into the burns. The prescription was sort of a placebo, for I was certain that as soon as he was able, he would lick it off. I demonstrated how to apply the ointment and asked them to put it on three times daily.

(When applying the medication, it would be necessary for them to observe the lesion. Thus they would be able to evaluate its progress.) I suggested that it might be best to keep their pet overnight so I could check him later, and the doctor in the morning could also check him before he sent him home. The Smyths assured me they were responsible owners. They would stay up and watch him this evening and apply the medication as I directed.

On the way home, I looked for a gas station. I should have filled up the tank earlier, but was negligent. It was past one in the morning and no stations on my route home were open for business. When I got home, I put a marker on the Mustang's steering wheel to remind me to get gas first thing in the morning.

"Dead tired" would have been an apt description of the way I felt. The house was dark and quiet. I slipped into the bedroom, sat down to take off my shoes, and the phone rang. I reached for the phone and so did Marna. When she saw me, I received a sleepy, "Glad you are home, honey," greeting. I didn't have the opportunity to even close my eyes, for I had to leave to attend another emergency at the Hawthorne hospital I had just left.

I dressed and went out to the Mustang. I saw my note on the steering column, and knew that I did not have enough gas to get there and home again, so I got Marna's keys from the kitchen and took her car.

The streets were empty so I was heavier on the accelerator than I realized—and had the same results as before! The reflection of a red light filled the interior of the car. I pulled over a couple of blocks from the previous location.

The same story as before: "May I see your driver's license, please." As I handed it to him, he gave me a long hard stare. Without cracking a smile, he said, "Thought you could fool me by changing cars, didn't you!" It was then that I realized I was talking to the same officer. He handed me back my license and said, "I know exactly what you are going to say. You are going to tell me that you are a dog doctor on the way to a hospital on an emergency." I could only grin. He asked me the location of the hospital and then informed me he was going to drive there obeying all the speed limits. I had better not arrive there before he did. He returned to his patrol car, and I headed for Hawthorne obeying all the speed limit signs.

My client was there waiting for me. A great big old gray tomcat was looking through the screen door of the cage at me. He had been in many wars. Battle scars were everywhere—on his face, on his ears, and on his neck. He definitely was the big cat on the block. Mike glared at me with his left eye—his right eye was swollen closed and tearing. I suspected that he had been in another fight and I was going to be treating a corneal lesion.

Mike was a very docile cat. I stroked his head and he started purring. Next I gently reflected his lower eyelid to get a glimpse of the cornea. This procedure was painful and Mike objected. Several drops of the optical anesthetic, opthaine, were put into the eye, and we waited a minute or two for it to take effect. A few more drops were again administered to be certain the tissue was insensitive.

There was no objection this time. The lower lid was rolled back to reveal the cornea. No abrasion was noted. I moistened a Q-tip with opthaine and proceeded to probe more deeply around the eye itself. As I investigated with more care around the commissures of the eye, one tiny awn came into view. I realized that I had now located a foxtail. I grasped the awn with the intent of gradually removing it from the eye. The awn broke off. It was now necessary to use the ocular retractor to open the eye more widely, thus enabling me to grasp the body of the foxtail. To do this, Mike was sedated. When the eye area was completely exposed, I understood why the awn had broken. The foxtail had embedded itself so deeply into the tissue that when I grasped the weaker awn, it broke off—it could not stand the strain. But soon I was holding my trophy.

The area where the foxtail had been removed was hemorrhaging badly. I treated the eye and placed a pack on it. Then pressure was applied using a temporary elastic bandage around Mike's head. By the time the business portion of the emergency case was completed, it was time to remove the bandage. The bleeding had stopped.

It was nearly three in the morning when I finally got into bed for a few hours of sleep. In the morning, I felt that I had been awake all night. I did manage to remember to gas up my Mustang on my way to work—thanks to the reminder I had left on the steering wheel.

—32—

FAT CAT

My date this evening was with Plop. I had treated Plop before in the daytime practice. Plop was a shorthaired black domestic cat that weighed twenty-six pounds. He was not a big cat—he was just a very obese cat. He had short legs and an oversized paunch, giving him the appearance of a sway-backed nag.

In Plop's previous trips to the hospital, I had encouraged the owners, the Stewarts, to control his diet and to force him to exercise. Other veterinarians had made this recommendation too. If all efforts to get him to exercise were to fail, I instructed the owners to at least put Plop's food in one corner of the room, his cat box in another corner, and his water dish in the third corner—he needed some type of movement. Unfortunately this suggestion did not work. He would eat and drink, but then he would leave his mess on the floor in an attempt to get to his litter box—it took him too long to reach that destination.

Plop was the cat's nickname. His original name was Blackie. His nickname seemed to describe him more completely. In order to walk, he had to get up on his tiptoes so his stomach would not drag on the floor. This required considerable effort, and he could only walk two or three feet at a time without resting. When he stopped to rest, he would "plop" on the floor. This sound could be heard from the adjoining room. Fatigue was a big problem. To get from one room of the house to another, he had to be carried.

135

Plop had another problem that was related to his obesity. His belly was bald, as all the hair had been rubbed off. The complaint this day was that he had a moist sore on his underside that would not heal. It could be described more appropriately as a bedsore or an ulcer. It was a challenge for me to figure out some way to relieve Plop's discomfort, for his belly was constantly in contact with the floor.

We rolled him over to scrutinize his underside. I decided to give his belly a surgical bath as the moisture there had dust and dirt adhering to it. The greatest problem was drying him off. I needed to put him in the dryer cage on a special rack that allowed air to pass under him. That helped some. I had Mrs. Stewart come to the rear of the hospital to assist me. We turned Plop over, and she kept him in that position while I used a hand blow-dryer to get his fur dry. An antibiotic ointment with a vanishing creme base was rubbed into the raw areas. I mentioned to the Stewarts that I didn't think he would lick it off. They laughed. They informed me that there was absolutely no way he could reach his stomach. I agreed.

The next thing to do was to find something to cover the lesion and protect it from further irritation. I got a section of a large stockingette, cut two holes for his front feet, rolled it over his head, and drew his two front feet through the holes. Next I rolled the stockingette down the rest of his body and over the lesion. At his rump, two more holes were cut so that his rear legs would fit through them. Now he had a complete outfit on! A gauze pad was put against the lesion and under the stocking for padding.

Mrs. Stewart asked if I had a marking pen, and I found one in the front desk. She proceeded to mark a large seven on each side of the stocking. "That" she said, "is my favorite number, and if we race him, I am certain he will win." We all had a good laugh, for we knew that a turtle could easily beat him in a race.

As I headed toward Palos Verdes for my next emergency call, I could not help but think of the story about the tortoise and the hare.

My clients had already arrived. They held a little puppy in their arms, and it had a one-pound coffee can stuck over its head. The owners had the foresight to punch a few holes in the bottom of the can, otherwise the pup would have suffocated. The can had some rough edges on it and could not be pulled off the pup's head. It also fit so snugly that there was no room for tin snips to be used. They thought they could snip the edges of the can and deflect them back so the rough portion would not be against the pup—then the pup's head could be easily removed. It was a good idea but could not be implemented. Between his wife giving him instructions and the pup whining and wiggling, both owners felt that it would be best for me to see him. I tried to cut the can with my tin snips but my effort was no better than that of the Stewarts.

In the treatment room I administered the short-acting anesthetic, surital. When all was quiet and I had time to think, I tried again with my tin snips. I was able to cut the can and deflected the edges. The can slid off easily. There were several minor scratches on the pup's head and neck, but those would heal nicely. The pup had been very fortunate. It was alive only because the owners had the foresight to punch holes in the can. With the can removed, the pup could now see which direction he was walking, and he could eat and drink as well.

Manhattan Beach was my next destination. It was nice to take emergencies there now, for they had just hired an all-night attendant. This person would not only assist me, but when an emergency arrived, he would make the entries on the patient card, and then, when I left, he would clean up the premises.

My client had already arrived and the attendant was completing the paperwork. The complaint from the Oakleys was that Tibet, their Llaso Apso, was constantly gagging. Sometimes he would gag so violently that he would spit up foamy blood. It had been going on for a couple of weeks, and could not be classified any longer as a passing circumstance—it was getting progressively worse.

Will, my evening's assistant, held Tibet careful while I examined his throat. The tonsillar area was slightly inflamed, but otherwise the throat appeared normal. The problem was likely to be deeper in the throat than I could see. A series of x-rays were taken. The view of the radiographs caused some concern, so a couple oblique views were taken. There was a very suspicious density about two inches down the esophagus on the left side. I went over the view with the owners and we discussed several possibilities. Finally we felt it best to anesthetize Tibet and search the throat in depth in order to make a more thorough exam.

It was necessary to work quickly. Intubating and using gas anesthetic was out of the question, for the endotracheal tube would be in the trachea and in the way. I inserted a fiberoptic scope into the esophagus and saw a foreign body of some kind. It was hanging down the throat on a cord or string. Using forceps, I was able to grasp it and deflect it into the mouth. It was a string with a knot on it. The string had cut its way underneath the tongue and then been overgrown by tissue. It could not be seen by an oral view. I cut the string and pulled it out by grasping the knot and pulling the string through the soft tissue. I gave an injection of chloramphenicol and had Will put Tibet in a cage.

I took the string out in front to show the Oakleys. They recalled how it might have happened. They were going to be gone for a few days so they gave Tibet the rest of the pork roast that they had for their evening meal. They didn't think to remove the string that tied the roast when it was offered to Tibet as a snack. The string had looped around under her tongue causing it to hang down into her trachea. She had been gagging since about the time they had returned from their trip.

While Will was cleaning up and I was still in conversation with the clients, another call came in. Will answered the phone and asked them to come right down. The Vances soon arrived with Willie, their Boston terrier. They were regular clients of the Manhattan hospital, so Will pulled the records when they arrived. We proceeded into the exam room.

Willie had been hit by a car, and it was evident that his right front leg was broken. X-rays were essential. It was not necessary to sedate Willie as he was still groggy from the trauma of the accident. Solu-delta-cortef was given intravenously for shock and a five-percent solution of saline and dextrose was administered slowly by IV drip as well. After shock treatment was initiated, several views were taken of the fractured leg. The fracture was a bad one and needed to be stabilized to avert further damage. It was a spiral fracture and several bone fragments were present. The olecranon of the elbow was also separated from the ulna. The leg needed to be protected so that the sharp edges of the bone did not lacerate or sever nerves, veins, or arteries.

A traction splint was fitted and the leg padded for extra protection. Will would monitor the case through the night, and in the morning the doctor would perform corrective surgery. The owners seemed to be relieved that Willie would be under supervision overnight. They were reminded to call in the morning and find out how their pet was doing. In the morning the doctor would discuss surgery and the expense involved.

I was able to head home as soon as the clients left. Will would do any further cleanup and call me if there were any questions about Willie. I called Marna and she asked me to pick up some Subway sandwiches on the way home. When I arrived, the boys were hungry and waiting. Marna had fixed root beer floats. We enjoyed the meal and talked about the danger of allowing pets out in the street where they could be harmed.

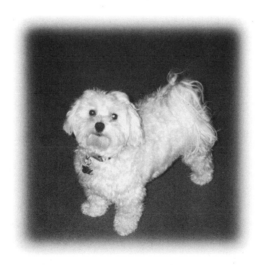

33

UNINVITED GUEST

It was Thursday evening when a friend from church called me directly and wanted to know if I had time to see their cat, Mimic. Mimic had swallowed a needle and thread. The thread was hanging out of her anus. When they applied light tension to the thread, Mimic would cry. The needle may have been there for two or three days, for her cat box did not have any stool in it for that period of time.

Marge and Bill Whitman met me at the Redondo Beach hospital. They had been concerned that a needle may be at the other end of the thread. When I checked Mimic, I agreed with their reasoning.

X-rays were taken to find the location of the possible needle. The radiograph indicated it was between two and three inches from the anus. The point of the needle was directed toward her head. I could easily see the eye of the needle due to a lucky positioning when the film was taken.

Surgery seemed imminent but I wanted to try something else first. As the needle was being dragged backwards, the head or eye end of the needle had become lodged in the wall of the rectum. If I could only repel the needle slightly there was a chance that I could recover it without extensive surgery.

A short-acting anesthetic was given, a tracheal tube passed, and Mimic was connected to the gas anesthetic machine. This would eliminate any straining during my recovery attempt. I tied a piece of surgical suture material to the short piece of exposed thread. Next I lubricated about a six-inch piece of half-inch rubber tubing. The thread with the suture material was passed through the tubing. The tubing now sleeved the thread and was passed through the anus very slowly. The tubing was teased into position and the needle was repelled ever so slightly because I did not want either end of the needle to penetrate the intestinal wall.

I applied slight tension to the thread. I could feel the needle moving against the tubing. A little more manipulation of the tube and the needle appeared at the exposed end of the tubing. The needle had been removed without making an incision!

The Whitmans were delighted. I was relieved not to have to do surgery. Bill said that it would be a great story to relate at the next Rotary luncheon, but I suggested that it was not really a mealtime subject.

Mimic was sent home in a half-awake/half-asleep state with instructions to give her half a teaspoon of mineral oil every four hours until she passed a normal stool.

My next call was at a nearby hospital. A Dalmatian named Fire had a badly swollen ear—probably from an insect bite. All of this was relayed to me by the answering service. I asked the operator to call the client and tell them that I would be at the hospital in twenty minutes.

Fire was brought into the examination room. His ear was so swollen that it was hanging out in a horizontal manner. It looked as if he was attempting to make a signal for a left turn. I helped lift him up on the table so I could get a better look at his ear. The problem was a blood-filled ear—a hematoma of the ear. (A hematoma is a blood blister—a pocket of blood under the skin. The origin of this problem is usually a foreign body in the ear or a trauma.) Fire could have had a foxtail in his ear and in his attempt to shake it out, hit his ear against an object, rupturing a blood vessel. Or the problem could have been simple—he may have just run into a corner of a building and pinched his ear between the building and his skull. In either case, the ear was full of blood and very annoying to him.

Two things needed to be done—the ear needed to be checked and the hematoma reduced. No foreign bodies were found in either ear. The hematoma was lanced and the blood removed from the ear. I made another small incision in the ear and then inserted a piece of plastic tubing, with holes cut in it like a French drain, into one incision of the ear and out the other. Then I anchored the tubing in place at each end. The ear was padded with gauze and the head wrapped to prevent blood from being scattered all over the place if he shook his head. The bandage would remain in place for a week and at that time could be taken off or replaced. I helped carry Fire out to the car and the clients were on their way home.

The answering services were called and none of them had any messages for me. I, too, headed for home. As I opened the back door of our house, the smell of popcorn and hot apple cider rushed out. We were able to spend the rest of the evening in what we called "family time." Each of us had the opportunity to tell what had happened to them during the day or week without anyone interrupting. We had the rule that each of the boys could only tell what he had done—not what his brothers had done. If one of the boys had something good or special to tell about his brother, he had to ask that brother for permission to do so. This policy resolved a lot of arguments and bad feelings before they had a chance to develop.

The next day was Sunday. After church and Sunday school, we dropped the boys off at a friend's house, and Marna and I went to a pool-side party in the peninsula hills. Our hosts had a beautiful home with an exquisite view. To the south we could see the harbor and the Pacific Ocean, and to the north we could see the lights of Los Angeles in the distance. About fifty guests were present and we visited around the pool. I was standing near the punch bowl when there was a commotion at the far side of the pool deck.

Guests were scattering and their voices conveyed concern. Soon I spied the problem. A skunk had emerged from the surrounding vegetation and it was walking around the pool. Everyone near it was giving it a wide berth. Others who were too near it when they first spotted it were standing stock-still as the varmint passed close by.

No one thought to close the sliding glass door of the house that separated the family room from the pool deck. Our black and white friend proceeded through the open door and went directly into the family room. He inspected the family room while the guests there stood like statues with their mouths open in disbelief. The skunk then walked over to the fireplace and curled up in the back corner and took a nap.

When the skunk had settled down, human activity commenced again. My friends began to chant, "Call the vet!" "Call the vet!" I was now a consultant!

I had no means of getting the skunk out of the fireplace and then out of the house. The situation presented a problem. If the skunk sprayed, the odor would be present for weeks. If any of his spray got on their champagne carpet, ink-like spots would appear when it dried. I thought that the host should call the Humane Society and see if one of their officers would come out and remove the skunk. The call was made. No officer was available because they were short staffed on that Sunday. Someone would be available in three or four hours.

Some encouragement had to be made that was enticing to the officer. I called this time. I introduced myself and asked if someone was available. I asked if they would connect me to that person. I was connected by radio. I explained the problem and made a fifty-dollar offer if he would come right away. Fifteen minutes later, he pulled into the driveway.

The owners wanted to get the skunk out of the house before he discharged. This Humane Society officer was an expert. The host found a half sheet of plywood in the garage and the face of the fireplace was blocked off. Next a huge piece of cotton was saturated with chloroform and tossed near the skunk.

Ten minutes later the plywood was tilted back to get a peek at the skunk. The skunk was well anesthetized. Gloved hands removed the skunk and deposited him in a cage. The cage was taken to the truck. The officer returned to take the plywood outside and the host handed him a crisp fifty-dollar bill. The guests applauded the officer as he left.

The skunk had been a frequent visitor to the neighborhood, but had never been so bold as to venture into a house before. The hostess had nicknamed the skunk "Cop" because he was black and white and occasionally showed up when least expected.

The events did teach the hostess a lesson. She was reminded that her cats should be fed inside. If they are fed outside, the food should be out of reach of opossums, raccoons, and skunks. Food is what attracts these critters and makes them unafraid of people.

—34—

SORE FEET

It was almost dusk when I took my fourth call. Most of the previous trips had been uncomplicated and of a "routine" nature. (No case was ever really routine, but each case was unique.) The call that I was responding to had all the earmarks of being unusual. It had a degree of urgency.

The emergency phone call came from the Palm Springs area, about one hundred miles away. The owners said that they could be at the Hawthorne hospital in about an hour and a half. "Would you meet me there?" was the question. I confirmed via the answering service that I would be there by that time.

I arrived a bit early. Suddenly tires screeched and a car pulled into the parking lot. Car doors slammed, and the front door of the hospital was flung open. The owner came bustling in, walked past me into the exam room, and placed his dog on the table. His only remark was that a terrible thing happened and his dog could not walk.

I decided to address the needs of the dog first, and then get the pertinent information from the owners later. The pads of the dog's feet were torn off—all four feet. The feet were bleeding and dirty. The dog's right shoulder was also raw and bleeding, and considerable hair and skin loss was evident all over the body. I went right to work. In the reception room, the wife and two children were crying.

I sedated the Labrador with surital while the owner restrained him. I asked the owner to wait in the reception room with his wife and his

144

children. The Lab was put on a rolling cart, taken into the treatment room, and connected to the metafane gas anesthetic machine machine that I had previously brought in from my car. An intravenous solution of isotonic saline was connected to the surital syringe that had been taped in place and a slow drip was started. Each foot needed to be debrided, cleaned, and sutured as needed. Then they were packed with furacin ointment and bandaged. (Furacin ointment is frequently used to treat burns as well as other exposed tissue.) Considerable hair needed to be clipped from various places over the dog's body to keep it from sticking to the moist areas and causing a problem. Each lesion was carefully scrubbed and treated according to its individual needs. The lesion on the shoulder was particularly severe, for the skin had been abraded almost down to the bone. A furacin pack was put there and then taped to the body. I stood back and looked at my patient—there were not many places on his body that had not received my attention. He looked as if he had been a war casualty.

I disconnected the Lab from the anesthetic machine. I went out front to the reception room and invited the family to come back to the treatment room with me to see their dog. They petted their dog and one of the children looked up at me and said, "CoCo will get well, won't he?" I assured the family that CoCo had a good chance now, but that it would take a long time for him to heal. They followed me into the ward and helped me lift CoCo from the rolling treatment table. The children got down on their knees and gave him more of their loving attention before all five of us returned to the reception room.

They had been clients at this hospital, and CoCo's medical record would be filed under the name "Brownell." I went down the list of previous entries—CoCo, chocolate in color, Labrador, male, five years old. When this was done, I looked at them and asked what happened. Mr. Brownell was the spokesman.

"We had spent the week in the desert and were returning home when we had a flat tire. The weather was hot so all of the family got out of the car—CoCo also. He decided to seek shade under the back of the car, so I tied him to the trailer hitch. We had to unload the trunk to get to the spare. When the tire was changed and all of the luggage returned to the trunk, I was hot and perspiring freely. I got a towel from the backseat to dry myself off and just got into the car and left. About a quarter mile down the highway, a car pulled up beside me and pointed behind the car. I didn't communicate with their gesture, so they rolled down their window and said something about a dog. I quickly pulled over. We had dragged CoCo almost a fourth a mile!"

From the lesions that I had just treated, I told them that CoCo must have run behind the car for a bit until he had lost his balance and fallen. He could not regain his balance due to the car speed and followed the rest of the way on his side until they were flagged down by the passing car. Then CoCo had then been bundled up and held on their children's laps. They had stopped at the first opportunity to phone.

They had had nothing to eat since their unfortunate incident, so while I had been treating their dog, Mrs. Brownell had walked down the street and purchased some drinks and sandwiches for all of us. We sat in the reception room and dined. We visited, and the children appeared to be much stronger emotionally. One more trip was made to the back of the hospital. CoCo raised his head when the family arrived and he even attempted to wag his tail. They were overjoyed at his response and this gave them considerable encouragement.

CoCo would remain at the hospital for several days. Both of the adults thanked me and the children each gave me a hug. I thanked them for the sandwich and the drink and they departed. How long CoCo remained in the hospital depended on the decision of their regular veterinarian. (Before the week was out, I had a thank-you note from one of the children. It included a sketch of me standing by the treatment table treating CoCo with captions under it saying, "Thank you, Doctor, for saving my dog's life.") All of this appreciation made me feel great!

After the Brownell family had left, I checked with Marna and she asked me to call the Torrance exchange. The Nelsons had called about their beagle female, Spot, who had a pendulous mammary tumor. The tumor had been there for some time. Recently it had been enlarging at an alarming degree. Now it was so large that occasionally it would strike the ground, causing an abrasion on its distal extremity.

We met at the hospital and Spot was lifted carefully to the exam table. The mass was indeed large, and extensive surgery would be required to remove it. Spot was ten years old, and her health had deteriorated notice-ably in the last couple of months. The Nelsons were at odds as to what to do and needed help in making a decision since Spot was an old dog.

I suggested that an x-ray be taken to see if the tumor had metastasized to any other parts of her system. I was particularly concerned about a radiograph of her lungs. If there were foci on her lungs, this cancer was definitely metastatic. Two views were taken and, indeed, multiple foci were evident in her lung tissue as I had expected.

A decision had to be made, for Spot's life would likely be downhill from now on. Each of the Nelsons gave Spot a hug and the necessary papers were signed. I took the beagle to the rear of the hospital and performed the necessary but undesirable task. The Nelsons had waited and they came to the back of the hospital to look at Spot for the last time.

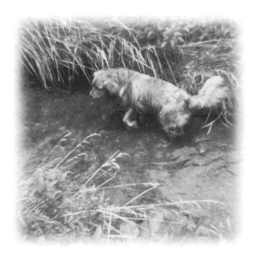

—35—

EXPERT WITNESS

It was Sunday morning and the children were just getting ready for church when I was called to the phone. A woman in Palos Verdes had injured a peacock and wanted me to see it. (Peacocks are a protected bird in the Palos Verdes Hills.) I never claimed to be proficient in avian medicine—probably because it was not of too much interest to me. However, as I cruised along in my Mustang on the way to this emergency, my thoughts were on how to treat a peacock.

(Peacocks are common in certain areas of the Palos Verdes Peninsula. They were first introduced into the area by the Vanderlips years ago. They are beautiful birds, but are very much a nuisance. At the crack of dawn, they wake the neighborhood up with their calling. During the day, they consume your flowers and anything else that appeals to them. Then to make matters worse, they mess all over your porches, driveways, and pool decks. The residents like to watch them, but prefer that the birds reside everywhere but in their own backyards.)

I needed to see this injured bird that I assumed had been hit by a car. I met the client in the parking lot and helped her remove the peahen from the car and then helped her get the bird into the exam room. It could not walk and appeared to be paralyzed. The peahen was taken into the x-ray room and two views were taken. I asked the client to step out of the room while the x-ray machine was on because she was obviously pregnant. When I brought the film out from the darkroom and positioned it on the view screen, I noted that the woman was irritated and showed little remorse for the injured bird. I shrugged off that observation and proceeded to show her the film. I then explained my findings. The peahen had a broken back. I suggested that it may have been hit by a car and that it was kind of her to bring it in for medical attention. It would be necessary to euthanize the bird so it would no longer suffer.

At this time the woman started crying. She said she didn't mean to do it. I didn't understand her comment, but assumed she had hit the peahen with her car. She explained what had happened.

Milk was delivered by the milkman to her back door in the typical glass bottles. She went out to retrieve the morning delivery and was attacked by this peahen. (A nest was later found nearby.) She was startled and dropped both milk bottles that broke when they came in contact with her concrete walk. Broken glass and spilled milk were everywhere. "I was infuriated. I grabbed a garden rake that was leaning against the side of the house and gave that darn peacock a healthy crack with it. It lay still after I hit it. Even after I cleaned up the mess, it still lay there. Then I felt bad for what I had done. I decided then that I had the responsibility to bring her in for you to fix up."

I sympathized about her misfortune, but again reassured her that there was nothing to do but to put the bird to sleep. An injection of pentabarbitol was given. The peahen was now dead.

The saga did not end at this point, for a couple of months later I had a call from the court to come in to the local magistrate's office and bring the radiographs with me. The woman who had hit the peahen was also present at this hearing. Someone had heard her story and reported her for killing a protected bird.

The views were shown and interpreted by me. My position was one of an expert witness. The woman told the story. The judge listened carefully and during the detailed rendition of the event remained stoic.

When all had a chance to speak, the judge stated that a fine needed to be levied for killing a protected species. "Before a fine is levied, is there any further testimony that needs to be submitted?" was the judge's remark. At this stage, I pointed out that technically I had killed the bird. My client had only injured it and was kind enough to take it to a hospital for care. "A point well taken," was his remark. He fined her twenty-five dollars.

I personally felt that many residents on the peninsula would gladly pay twenty-five dollars a bird to rid the neighborhood of the destruction they caused. I understood the spontaneous reaction of the woman and it was kind of the judge to levy such a minimal fine.

(Peacocks are not afraid of cats and will approach them with their feathers unfurled as they do when they strut. Cats will back off and duck for cover. Dogs are different—they are more aggressive. Almost any size dog will chase a peacock until it flies out of their yard. When this happens, the problem of peacocks and their messes are passed on to the next-door neighbor. Peahens become very protective when they nest or have little ones in the area.)

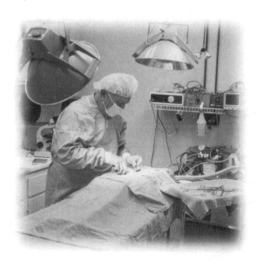

—36—

PICNICKING WITH
PATIENTS

Saturday day shifts often enabled me to get home early. Rarely did any hospitals stay open past three in the afternoon. The day was bright and sunny, and my plan, for the late part of the afternoon, was to sit out in the backyard, soak up some sunshine, and watch the sun ebb in the west with a cold drink at my side. This would be more pleasurable than working in the yard.

As I turned off the ignition on the Mustang, the boys rushed out to greet me. All were talking at once. I held my finger to my lips—this was a prearranged quiet sign that Marna and I had introduced in order to hear phone conversations. It worked! The boys were suddenly silent. I asked Allen what was going on. George responded, "Mom is planning a picnic."

A picnic had not been part of my plans for the afternoon, but soon I was inside changing into clothes appropriate for the occasion. Too many times Marna had scheduled something only to have my emergency cases interrupt those plans. It was still early in the day and I realized that some of my "spare time" should be spent with my family. This would be a special afternoon.

We loaded one car with all of the picnic supplies—food, blankets, and folding chairs. At the last minute, I returned to the garage and added two lounge chairs to our other car. We waved to Greta as we pulled out of the driveway in our separate cars, and she gave us a plaintive bark, as if to say "Why am I being left at home?"

Since we were heading to the Torrance park, we had to drive by the Torrance hospital where I had worked that morning. There was a case there that I needed to check on, and there was no time like the present, so we both stopped and I went inside. The surgical case was doing fine— she was walking back and fourth behind the cage door just begging to get out. As I returned to the parking lot, a car pulled in beside ours.

The driver asked if I was a veterinarian. I said, "Yes." I wasn't dressed professionally, so the client wanted to be certain. They had a pet in distress in their car and wanted me to come over to their car and take a peek at her. Instead, I asked them to bring their dog into the hospital so I could examine her properly. They put a leash on her and followed me. Allen was with me, so he held the front door open and directed the Brinkleys toward the examination room. They placed their Weimaraner, Babe, on the table. Babe was indeed in distress. Her abdomen was very swollen. Mr. Brinkley said, "We might have a case of bloat here in Babe. I have seen this many times on my dad's dairy farm." I concurred that their dog was very bloated, but I could not determine the cause without taking an x-ray. We carried Babe into the x-ray room and then took the necessary views of the abdomen. I confirmed the diagnosis of a gastric torsion.

Surgery was necessary and it had to be done soon. Allen wanted to stay and help me, so I had him go out to the car and tell his mother to go on to the park in her car and we would meet her there later. The Brinkleys agreed to the surgery in order to save Babe's life. I was not familiar with this surgical technique for corrective surgery. I called Carl, a colleague, to come in and do the surgery while I assisted.

Marna came in to inquire how long the surgery would take. I told her about two hours after Carl arrived. I heard a frustrated sigh as she left the hospital and returned to her car. Allen then agreed to go on to the park with his brothers.

I set up surgery while Carl was on his way. The Brinkleys asked what would cause this type of problem. I tried relating the sequence of events that likely led to this type of obstruction, but had no success. They didn't understand so I decided to demonstrate. I placed a weight in some tubular stockingette and flipped it around while holding each end. This motion would strangulate both the entrance to the stomach and the exit from the stomach. I told them that this is what likely had happened. Babe ate a lot of food at one time, probably dry food, and then consumed a quantity of water. This provided the weight. Afterwards she was playing vigorously and somehow the stomach rotated.

The Brinkleys looked at each other and Mrs. Brinkley said, "That could well be. I saw Babe drink water after she ate and then we threw a ball to her for awhile. Babe finally got tired and went over to lay down. She had never quit like this before, but I never thought much of it. Later Wes came in and said that Babe was standing in an awkward position and moaning."

Carl came in at this time. The Brinkleys decided to wait in the front room, so Carl and I proceeded with surgical preparations. We sedated her, put her on an intravenous drip, and connected her to the anesthetic machine. We were now ready for surgery.

Carl made the midline incision and exposed the stomach. The next thing that we had to do was to relieve the bloat and then remove the ingesta from the stomach. When this was done, we closed the gastrotomy incision and then turned our attention to correcting the rotation of the stomach. This was the most complicated part of the surgery, and, between the two of us, the alignment of the stomach was returned to normal. A retention suture from the stomach to the body wall was put in so the stomach would remain in the correct position. Closure was completed. Babe was disconnected from the anesthetic machine. We changed the fluid drip by connecting a new bottle of saline and dextrose. We removed our gloves—surgery was over.

While we were stepping out of the surgery room, I heard the front door open. Expecting another client, I went to the reception room, but found the Brinkleys reentering. They had decided to step out for a bite to eat rather than pace the floor at the hospital. In their hands were burgers and drinks for both Carl and me. I thanked them and then sat down with the Brinkleys and talked through the surgical procedure we had done. Carl took the sandwich and drink with him as he headed home.

After the Brinkleys had purchased the food, they had driven over to the Torrance park to eat it. "We parked right next to your wife's car," he said. "We recognized her and your oldest son right away. I even played some catch with the boys while my wife visited with yours."

I obtained a deposit from them and told them I would call later so they would be informed about Babe's recovery. Mrs. Brinkley said, "Your wife told me to tell you that they would wait for you at the park." After the

Brinkleys left, I took what was left of my sandwich and coke and headed for the park.

Marna's timing was perfect. Blankets had been spread out on the grass and the picnic was ready for immediate consumption. The boys were milling around waiting for me. We sat down in a circle and held hands. I said grace and thanked the Lord for the beauty that surrounded us and for the opportunity to sit down as a family and partake of His bounty.

We finished the late lunch. I glanced at the nearest lounge chair with a plan of utilizing it while the boys played. Marna was picking up the remains of the meal and stowing it in the cool box. I didn't quite make it to the chair. The boys had other ideas. They escorted me out on the grass to play some catch with them. By now Marna had completely packed everything in her car except one lounge chair. I thought it was for me, but when I glanced over again, she was well settled in it watching us play catch and also admiring the red and orange sunset.

It was the third of July and on Sunday the nation would celebrate the Fourth of July. The sun had completely set on the horizon when we got home. We returned all of the picnic supplies that were in Marna's car to their proper paces when the phone rang. A client was desperate. Tomorrow was the Fourth of July and he had forgotten to refill his tranquilizer prescription for his Doberman. Doby had gone crazy last year with all of the fireworks—especially the noisy ones. Last year he had jumped through the front door screen and disappeared for three days. Doby was later apprehended by the Humane Society and Mr. Claibourne had to pay a fine to get him out of jail.

He wanted to meet me at any hospital of my choice and pick up the necessary prescription. He was not a client of any of the hospitals that I was associated with. I would thus be unable to refill a previous prescription. That was okay—he just wanted me to prescribe what was needed anyway.

I sympathized with his problem. I explained that Doby needed to be checked physically before I would send home any medication. That was the law. He felt that that procedure was stupid, but when he realized that I was holding fast to my reason, he agreed to meet me at the closest hospital with Doby.

When I got through checking Doby and filling the prescription, I presented Mr. Clairbourne with the charges. He noted that I did not charge for an examination. I smiled and said that I was not required to charge an office visit—only to examine my patient to comply with the law. Mr. Clairbourne broke into a broad grin. He shook my hand, then said, "You vets are not as money conscious as I suspected."

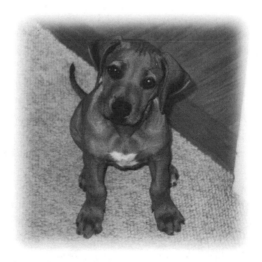

37

DOG GONE

The Fourth of July had rolled around again. In fact, it had passed and it was now the eighth of July. The call from the Palos Verdes hospital was about a problem that was initiated on the holiday. I was asked if I would talk to the owner who was on the line. I agreed. Butch belonged to the Collins family. "Butch had been missing since firecrackers had been going off last Sunday. He had been hiding in the garage, but that is a long story. Butch has not had food or water for probably five days. He is dehydrated and I just want you to check him over."

Mrs. Collins was with Butch in the parking lot when I arrived. She was trying to walk him, but he just stood in one spot and trembled. She picked up her wire-haired terrier and followed me into the hospital. I directed her to go into the examination room while I pulled Butch's records from his home hospital's file cabinet. Butch was still trembling when I entered the exam room. Was he shaking because of his previous experience or was he just responding to my presence?

Butch was an older dog and noise greatly disturbed him. I checked him over and could perceive nothing adverse other than a rather severe dehydration—his skin was not as pliable as it should have been. I drew a blood sample and put it into the centrifuge. The packed cell volume was higher than normal indicating a loss of body fluids.

I thought that when his hydration returned to normal that he would probably feel much better. As he had not eaten very much since he was found, I suggested that a liter of five-percent saline and dextrose given intravenously would probably be the most beneficial for his recovery. I rolled in an IV drip stand and hung a bottle of the solution from it. Mrs. Collins held Butch while I established the drip. I then secured the needle and tubing in place by taping it to his front leg. Mrs. Collins agreed to hold Butch while the fluid was being administered. I regulated the drip to one drop every four seconds. Now it was time for me to pause.

Mrs. Collins said, "You will never believe what happened. We store an old mattress in the gable of the garage. When all the fireworks were going off, somehow Butch got up on the car and then up on the mattress in the garage where he would be safe from all of the noise. I took the car out of the garage late on the fourth when I went shopping. When I returned, I parked in the driveway to unload the groceries. If the weather is nice, I sometimes leave the car out of the garage for days.

"About a couple of hours ago I left on an errand and when I returned, I decided to park my car in the garage. When I turned off the engine and was removing the keys from the ignition, Butch jumped down from above. He scared me to death. He was shaking and so was I. I gathered him up and took him inside. I offered him food and water. He refused the food and took only a lap or two of water. He just stood there looking at me and trembling. I was worried and thought he should be seen right away. Quite a story, isn't it?"

I could only shake my head as Mrs. Collins related the circumstance to me. Butch was beginning to show some improvement. He had stopped trembling. I know that the intravenous feeding helped, but I think that standing by his master's side probably had a greater healing effect.

I opened a can of dog food and offered some to him. He turned his head and ignored me. Mrs. Collins took a little from the can in her hand and Butch accepted it. He ate about one-fourth of a can in this manner before I stopped him. It was not good for him to eat too much solid food at one time.

Butch was disconnected from the venous feeding when the liter bag was empty. I sent the rest of the canned food with Mrs. Collins and two more cans of the high-protein diet with the instructions to give him only a little at a time. Also, if she could encourage him to drink, it would help him immensely. She picked up Butch and walked out the door. As she left the premises, there was Butch licking the side of her face and his tail was constantly in motion.

I checked with Marna and she asked me to call the Hawthorne hospital's exchange. Miss Martin had just gotten home and found that her rabbit and cat—both which had the run of the house—had had a disagreement. Her cat had mauled Ears, the rabbit. Her cat had bitten and scratched Ears and the bunny had squeezed itself under the couch out of reach of the cat's claws.

Miss Martin and Ears arrived. His ears had been bitten and there were puncture wounds in many places over his entire body. It looked as if the cat had carried him around and played with him. Ears had probably escaped several times only to be caught and taken out to an open spot in the room and released for another game of "catch the rabbit."

I decided against clipping the rabbit's fur to treat the multitude of puncture wounds. I put antiseptic solution on all the wounds that I could locate and then advised her to brush the rabbit twice daily to keep the fur from matting over the lesions. I then made up some liquid ampicillin and showed her how to give it orally to Ears. I said, "You will be very experienced when all the treatment is over because I want you to give the antibiotic solution three times daily—in the morning, when you get home from work, and just before you retire."

Miss Martin took care of the charges and headed for the door. I stopped her. I explained that the cat and the rabbit would have to be kept apart at all times or this would happen again. "Even if you are home, don't trust your cat to leave Ears alone—the next encounter could be fatal." She looked up at me with tear-filled eyes and said, "I will have to get rid of one of them, but I don't know if I can make the choice!"

As I cleaned up the hospital, I noticed a note on the bulletin board with my name on it. It was from the Wallaces—the owner of Ginger, the Irish setter who had had the terrible skin problem. It read: "Doctor, even though you made us angry when you informed us we were grossly negligent concerning the care of our dog, Ginger, we agreed to follow your instructions if for no other reason than to prove you were wrong. We fed Ginger a high-protein diet and bathed her as you recommended. Her skin is much better and her improvement can be measured weekly. The best part is that we have established a routine for her care. The arrangement we made with you has been satisfied and we thank you for being so firm with us regarding Ginger's care." Signed: Alice Wallace.

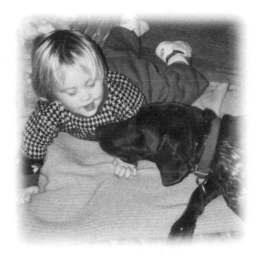

38

MY ASSISTANT

I had just hung up the phone after talking to Mrs. Womack about her cat with an injured tail when the phone rang again. This was an emergency call from a Mrs. Smyth whose cat had just been hit by a car. These calls were from different hospitals and the second call was the most urgent. I called Mrs. Womack back and asked her to meet me in about an hour at the Torrance hospital. I took Mrs. Smyth's call first at Redondo Beach.

The Smyth's cat, Snookums, was in bad shape. Snookums's anus was dialated and no sensation was evident when I manipulated its tail. In fact, the tail was as limp as a piece of wet rope. I walked down the spinal column carefully with my fingers and could palpate a distinct malalignment of the spinal cord in the lumbar area. There was a distinct dyspnea as the chest was heaving. From auscultation with the stethoscope, I heard distinct intestinal sounds in the thoracic area.

Snookums had been hit very hard by the car. My preliminary examination suggested both a broken back and a diaphragmatic hernia, let alone less evident problems.

I looked up at Mrs. Smyth and I guess she could read my expression. She asked how bad Snookums was injured. I told her what I suspected. The hernia probably could be mended, but the broken back probably meant that she would have paralysis in her hind quarters with the loss of both fecal and urinary function.

160

I waited a moment or two while she composed herself. She dried the tears from her eyes, and said, "Would you put her out of her misery?" I said, "Yes."

Mrs. Smyth settled her account. I put Snookums to sleep and then cleaned up in a hurry before heading to the Torrance hospital to take care of Mrs. Womack and her cat with the tail injury.

I was a few minutes late and found Mrs. Womack waiting with Partner. I went over to the Womack car and apologized for being late. She assured me that all was fine and asked if the other kitty was okay. I informed her that it had a broken back and had to be euthanized. "What a shame," was her response. She started to get her cat carrier out of the car so I assisted her and carried it into the hospital.

I filled out the medical record for Partner and we proceeded into the exam room. Mrs. Womack assisted Partner out of her cage. I immediately noted that she was dragging her tail.

Mrs. Womack explained that she did a lot of knitting, most of it sitting in her rocking chair while watching television. Partner had sat down beside her for a little affection. He then lay down and somehow got his tail under the rocker. "I felt the runner roll over his tail," she said. "He also let out a terrible cry and ran for his basket in the kitchen. I put down my knitting and followed him. There he was in his basket, licking his tail. I picked him up and gave him some love and looked at his tail closely. It was not bleeding, but it distinctly was out of line."

Only the tip of Partner's tail had been injured—the last two or three coccygeal vertibrae seemed to be involved. I remarked that technically Partner had a broken back. "Just like that other kitty you had just seen," she remarked. "Not exactly," was my response. "Partner's injury is in a very different location on the spine."

An x-ray was taken and two of the vertibrae had been crushed. My suggestion was to remove the injured portion of the tail. "It will hardly be missed," I said. Mrs. Womack agreed. "Make it short enough so that this misfortune will not be repeated," she jokingly said.

I suggested that Partner stay the night so we could evaluate aftercare. If he paid attention to his tail, we would bandage it—otherwise no bandage would be required. Mrs. Womack left and I went to work on Partner.

Halfway through surgery the phone rang, but I was unable to answer it. I did step into the treatment room to see which line the incoming call was on. It was the back line ringing indicating that it was either Marna or the answering service trying to reach me. I took off my gloves when the surgery was completed and called Marna. It was another emergency at the Redondo Beach hospital—a hamster problem of some nature. I asked Marna to call the service back and have them tell the client that I was forty minutes away and to meet me then.

When I arrived at the Redondo Beach hospital, no car was present in the parking lot. I didn't think that I would arrive there first, but went into the hospital through the back door. Then I unlocked the front door and noticed a bicycle leaning against the wall. Next to the bike was a young lady holding a wire basket with a hamster inside. We went into the hospital. Angie, the young lady, was crying. She had taken her pet hamster, Friday, out of his cage to let him play on the front lawn. A strange cat had come along and pounced on him and tried to carry him off. Angie had run after the cat, and the cat dropped Friday before it jumped the fence and disappeared.

Angie was the one that really needed attention. Friday only had a few bite wounds on his neck, and did not seem to be badly injured. If he was in shock, he did not show the symptoms. Angie, however, needed to be comforted and reassured that her pet would survive.

She held Friday while I checked him thoroughly. I carefully clipped the fur around each wound. During this process, I tried to distract Angie by asking questions.

"How far away do you live?" I asked.

"About four blocks."

"What grade in school are you?"

"Fourth grade."

"That makes you about ten, doesn't it?"

"I'm eleven now."

Angie was slowly regaining her composure and was of great assistance to me. We checked Friday carefully. Angie was far more observant than I. She would say, "Here's a bite mark, Doctor!" Then, "Here's another one!" Even though I was very careful in my inspection, I did not find as many bite marks as Angie. It was surprising what a pair of young eyes can see.

When Angie and I finished, Friday looked as if moths had gotten into his coat. Angie was smiling now that her pet was past any crisis. We put Friday back in his cage and went to the front desk. Angie handed me a five-dollar bill and said, "It's all I have, but I'll pay you the rest later." I did not accept her offer. I told her if she would clean off the exam table and help me put the instruments away, we would call it even. After all, I usually have all my assistants on the payroll. Angie wiped the exam table clean. I brought in the vacuum to pick up the clipped fur. She insisted on doing the vacuuming also.

Angie thanked me two or three times and gave me a special hug. I watched her peddle down the street with the hamster cage in her bicycle basket. What a privilege it was for me to help such a sweet youngster.

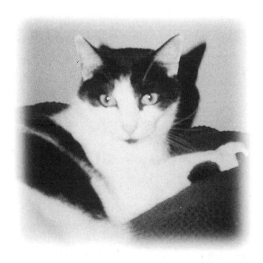

—39—

A DRY LITTER BOX

When a client called with the intent of only asking a question, and I recognized it as a bona fide problem, it was my responsibility to try to initiate an emergency call. Such was the case that I was responding to. Mrs. Scott called about her male cat, which was spending a good bit of his time in the cat box. However, there had not been any evidence of moisture in the box now for two days. Mrs. Scott's initial question was, "Do you think that Peco is urinating somewhere else in the house?"

This question suggested a urinary blockage problem often not recognized by a client. When a male cat spends a lot of time meditating in the cat box with no evidence of results, a real problem is in progress.

"Peco should be seen soon," I said.

"Can it wait until morning?"

"It would be best to see Peco tonight in case he has a urinary blockage. We certainly would not want the bladder to rupture."

"I'll take my child over to the neighbors and be at the hospital in thirty minutes."

"Great! I'll be waiting for you."

I finished dinner and headed for the Torrance hospital. I parked my Mustang and was unlocking the front door when Mrs. Scott arrived with Peco.

Peco was brought into the exam room. He was straining even when being held by his owner. I palpated the abdomen and the bladder was huge

164

in size—almost the size of a baseball. It was a serious problem and at a critical stage. I explained what needed to be done to correct the problem, and Mrs. Scott decided to wait. Her child was being taken care of and there was now no rush on her part. She asked to borrow the phone and inform her neighbor that she would be at the hospital for awhile.

Peco was sedated, entubated, and put on the gas anesthetic machine which I had just brought in from the Mustang. The anesthetic allowed me to try to pass a catheter, and since he would not be able to strain while sedated, he could not voluntarily resist my back-flushing technique.

(Sediment accumulates in the male cat's urethra at a point just anterior to the cartilage of the penis. When too much of it accumulates at one time, it packs tightly enough so that urine cannot pass, thus forming a complete block. A syringe full of saline attached to a special catheter is used to back-flush this sediment into the bladder. This usually enables the urine to flow freely again and some of the sediment is expelled in normal urination.)

The water pressure from my syringe was greater than the bladder pressure and the sediment was flushed back into the bladder. Blood-tinged urine began to flow from the end of the catheter. The bladder wall had been stretched to such a degree that some of the blood vessels had ruptured and blood was now mixed with the urine. Over sixty milliliters of blood-tinted urine was collected.

The most crucial part, the emptying of the bladder, had been accomplished. The next problem that concerned me was the tone of the bladder wall muscles. (Sometimes the bladder muscles are abused so much by overextension that they lose their capability of contracting. This means that the bladder would fill again but that the tomcat would not be able to urinate on his own. Either the urine continues to drip [urinary incontinence] or the sediment in the bladder could accumulate again and block the urethra as before. If the bladder loses its tone, the tomcat is no longer a desirable household pet. To determine if the bladder tone has been preserved, a urinary catheter is sutured in place and the cat remains in the hospital for several days. During this period of hospitalization, urine drips out of the catheter. The bladder wall now has a chance to rest and recover from it stretched condition.)

I took the beaker full of bloody urine out to show to Mrs. Scott and explained the cause of the hematuria. I discussed my recommendations and my prognosis concerning the case. Sometimes a pneumocystogram (radiograph of air-filled bladder) can provide vital information about the damage that has been done. The morning doctor could want to do this if he felt it of value.

"Can you do this now?"

"Yes, I can. It may be easier to do now that Peco is sedated."

Mrs. Scott remained in the reception room and I returned to the treatment room. To make my task easier, I reconnected Peco to the anesthetic machine before he woke up completely.

I carefully inflated the bladder with air using a large syringe connected to the catheter. When the bladder was fully inflated, I clamped off the catheter so that the air would not escape while I took the x-ray. A thin but uniform bladder wall was evident and no bladder stones were noted. I had previously saved a sample of the urine as well as one of the sediment to send to the laboratory for analysis. The doctor in the morning would call the lab and have them pick up the specimens. The laboratory report would be back before Peco was discharged and the doctor would know exactly what medication to dispense with Peco when he was discharged.

Mrs. Scott left the required deposit. I asked her to call her regular doctor daily for a progress report since Peco would be taking up residence at the hospital for several days. I related to her that I felt that she was very lucky to have an indoor cat or she never would have noted his problem.

We talked awhile about pet management at home and I expressed the need to watch the pet's intake of food as well as if it was eliminating properly. (Small amounts of food should be given at a time—just enough for one feeding—then you know if your pet is eating. If a food dish is kept full all of the time and a pet is allowed to "pasture" on it, there is no way to determine how much or if any is ever consumed. The same thought applies to a cat box. If the box is emptied daily, then that gives the owner an opportunity to note if the cat is eliminating properly.) "Peco is very fortunate that you are an observant owner," I told Mrs. Scott. We went on discussing the pros and cons of pet management when the phone rang.

I excused myself for a moment and answered it. Another case was on my agenda. An emergency at the Manhatan Beach hospital required my presence. I had to be on my way shortly. Mrs. Scott obliged by leaving and allowing me to clean up, put all the instruments away, bring Peco's medical record up-to-date, and head to my next destination.

Mrs. Wiggins arrived with her cat, Toots, who had just had a skirmish with her neighbor's dog. I filled out the medical record for Toots and then ushered both Mrs. Wiggins and Toots, who was in a cat carrier, into the examination room. Toots was "wired"—she was still bright-eyed and bushy-tailed. She was on edge and wary of my every move. A patch of skin was loose on her rump, but that did not appear to be bothering her at this moment. She was worried about her surroundings and as tense as a coiled spring.

Mrs. Wiggins had witnessed the accident. Toots roamed the neighborhood most of the time. The neighbor's dog was usually confined, but on occasion he got out and surveyed the neighborhood for something to chase. He was a large playful dog who ran after anything that would run from him. One of his favorite challenges was chasing Toots. Toots would head down the street with the intention of seeking safety behind a wrought-iron gate. She could get through the spokes of the gate easily, but the dog was restricted. When she knew she was safe, she would stop on the safe side just out of reach of the dog and just sit there and preen herself. She would wash her face using the sides of her moist paws and then just look at the dog and tease him.

All usually went well, but this time she made a mistake—she misjudged her safe distance just inside the gate. She was too close. The dog reached through the gate and grabbed at her, tearing a piece of skin on her backside.

We got Toots out of the cage. I checked the lesion. The patch of loose skin was in the shape of an inverted "L" and that was good, for vascular circulation runs down an appendage. This meant that the patch of skin was likely to be viable.

I doped up Toots with a short-acting anesthetic. Antibiotic powder was puffed into the wound, the hair was clipped, and I was ready to start suturing. The corner was sutured first to align the rest of the tissue. Then both sides were closed. Almost fifteen stitches were required to complete the closure of the wound.

I padded the carrying cage with a towel after I had administered antibiotics. Toots was able to go home now. I suggested that she remain in the cage until she desired to get out. We agreed on an appointment time in two weeks for suture removal. I reminded Mrs. Wiggins to keep a close watch on the incision line to see that Toots was leaving her stitches alone.

—40—

A MOUSE IN
THE HOUSE

As I left my daytime practice and stepped outside to my Mustang, I realized that it was getting dark much earlier than usual that evening. Ominous clouds were rolling in from the west and blocking the usual sunset that was a common sight for me. The air seemed so quiet. There was a vacuum feeling that surrounded me—no wind, no circulation. Only big black billowy clouds were gathering and slowly moving in to surround the south bay in their whispery arms.

Halfway home I found it necessary to turn on the headlights. I was remiss in not doing it earlier. The lights were on at home, and when I walked into the kitchen, Marna said that the weatherman had predicted a stormy night. It was dark as we sat down for dinner, and the boys felt that something mysterious was about to happen.

After supper, Marna and I stood on the front porch watching the storm clouds gather. The wind had picked up and was gusting. Lightening could be seen in the far distance as it illuminated the sky—this was a rare occurrence in southern California. Distant rumbles of thunder followed each illumination in the sky. The weather was taking on the profile of a good old-fashioned midwest thunderstorm. Marna said that she was going inside because she had felt some isolated drops of rain hit her bare arms. I did not stay on the porch very much longer either, for the misty rain had turned into large drops and then commenced to come down in torrents.

The boys had prepared the fireplace and soon the flickering light of the fire provided warmth to the family room. I felt reasonably secure that it would be unlikely I would have any reason to venture out that evening as no clients were likely to want to be out in this type of weather either.

I sat down in my leather chair by the fireplace and was reading to Albert when the lights dimmed, flickered, and then went out altogether. At the same moment, the phone rang. The service connected me with Mrs. Gibbons. Her kitten of four months of age had injured its front leg and she requested medical attention.

I donned some rain gear and left. The wind was really gusting now and it was blowing and raining so hard that the windshield wipers were not doing the job I expected of them. Caution was on my mind as I drove to the Palos Verdes hospital. The few cars that were on the road that blustery evening were driving cautiously as well. Forty-five minutes later I arrived and shortly Mrs. Gibbons and her two daughters pulled in and scurried into the hospital with their pet. Their kitten, Barbie, was confined in a cardboard box that had holes punched in it. Fortunately the electrical power was on in this area. The container was carried in by the older daughter, Susan. Jenny followed closely by her side and was constantly giving her older sibling instructions about how to carry the box—"don't tip it," "set it down gently," "keep your hands off the holes so Barbie can see out," etc.

Barbie indeed had an injured front leg. She objected whenever I touched it and cried when I rotated it. It was necessary to take a radiograph, so the family waited in the front room while I took Barbie to the rear of the hospital and took a picture of her left front leg.

When the film was developed, I took it to the exam room and placed it on the viewing screen so we could all look at it together. We carefully looked at the fracture. It was difficult for the girls to see the break because it was not too evident. I was looking at a green-stick fracture of the ulna about midshaft. There was a distinct crack in the ulna, but not a complete separation.

I told them that a green-stick fracture is more like a crack in the bone and it is the easiest type to protect and correct. All that needed to be done was to style a walking splint to accommodate the tiny leg. A young animal's bones heal rapidly so in a couple of weeks the splint could be removed if no further pain could be elicited.

"How did it happen?" I asked.

Jenny volunteered, "Susan did it!"

Mrs. Gibbons intervened and said, "It was an accident. Barbie caught a mouse outside and brought it into the house when we let her in. She wanted to brag about her accomplishment so she released the mouse on the kitchen floor for all of us to see. The mouse was not dead yet and it started running around the room with Barbie trying to recatch it. Finally I established order in the kitchen. All three of us were armed with yard-sticks and brooms and as Barbie chased the mouse around trying to play with it, we would take a swipe at the mouse with our weapons. Susan landed the fatal blow. She whacked the mouse, but also Barbie's leg with her stick. I picked up the mouse with a paper and laid it to rest in the garbage can outside.

"When I returned to the kitchen. Barbie was limping and not putting any weight on her foot. I tried to look at her foot, but she objected. I knew then that some damage must have been done. I am glad it was not a bad break. David, my husband, gets home late tonight from a business trip, and I promised the girls that they could stay up and tell their father this cat and mouse story."

Mrs. Gibbons wanted to borrow the film to show her husband the frac-ture, but I suggested an alternative. I went outside in the rain and cut a branch off of one of the bushes at the side of the hospital. I took it inside and bent it until it started to break. I then handed it to Susan. "Show this to your father and tell him this is what happened to Barbie's leg." We agreed that this was a good training aid and would certainly simplify the description of the fracture.

I got home and the electricity was still off. Marna had lighted an antique kerosene lamp and the boys were trying to find out which batteries in their flashlights would wear out first. They were playing the beams of the flashlights around the room in the manner that a searchlight searches the sky. Sleeping bags were strewn around the family room floor in front of the fireplace. Faux Pas was curled up near the hearth soaking up the heat and Greta was snuggled in between George and Albert. With the boys well settled for the rest of the night, Marna and I sat together on the couch with a steaming cup of coffee, watching the fire and observing the flashlight beams traverse the walls and ceiling.

The ring of the telephone disturbed the peacefulness that we were enjoying in the family room. I had not expected a single call on this stormy night and now I probably had two. I soon was talking to the Nicholses.

Another young pet was involved. It was a puppy. This poodle had been purchased two weeks ago. He was moping around the house and did not seem to have the vigor expected of a pup. Both husband and wife worked and they preferred bringing the pup in for an examination this night rather than take time off from work. I agreed to meet them at the San Pedro hospital and soon I was on my way again that rainy night.

The Nicholses arrived with Rocky. The pup looked unthrifty and showed none of the expected energy of youth. Rocky's temperature was normal. I positioned the stethoscope over his heart and could not distinguish a clear heartbeat. What I heard was more of a surging sound—a machinery murmur. This indicated a congenital heart defect. More technically it is called a patent ductus arteriosis, which is a shunt between the aorta and the pulmonary artery.

The Nicholses had purchased a defective pup. I asked them if they had thought of having a veterinarian examine the dog when they purchased it. "No," was their answer. "What kind of contract did you sign when Rocky was purchased?" They could not remember. My next course of action was to write a letter to "To whom it may concern" indicating that the pup had a congenital defect. The Nicholses were fond of their poodle and wanted to keep him. When I told them that it would not have a normal life and likely would die at an early age, they concurred with my advice.

I recommended that they return Rocky to the breeder and ask for a full refund. I did not recommend that they exchange him for any other pup in the litter (not a good idea to do when a defect that is hereditary is found). I told them that if the breeder did not agree with my diagnosis to have the breeder accompany them to a different veterinarian for another opinion. I was certain that my diagnosis would be confirmed. To get their investment back, it was necessary for the Nicholses to proceed in this manner.

I agreed to type a letter explaining my diagnosis to facilitate the recovery of their investment. I assured them that the letter would be available the next day at that hospital. They left in the pouring rain. As they were exiting the door, they were already discussing the possibility of finding another pup in the near future.

—41—

WHERE ARE THE KITTENS?

Emergencies can happen anywhere and at any time—sometimes even next door. Marna had seen Misty many times in the neighborhood. Misty had a daily route. She was expected to walk down our fence in the late morning, jump from the fence onto our brick barbecue, and disappear into the vegetation as she ventured into yet another neighbor's yard. This was almost her daily schedule, but Misty was not quite as mobile with the extra weight she was packing around now—she was very pregnant.

Misty did not perform her routine for several days. Marna thought she had delivered her kittens. That evening the doorbell rang and Misty's owners asked if we had seen her. We hadn't. I suggested that Misty had hidden her kittens somewhere she felt that they would be safe. The owners said that it was not likely, for Misty normally queened (gave birth) at home.

The next evening there was a knock on our door. Mrs. Crail was standing there with Misty in her arms. Misty had come home to eat. She was starved as well as very dehydrated. She wanted me to help her find where she had hidden her kittens. Together we reasoned that if we turned her loose at night, we could not visually track her. The most sensible thing to do was to feed her and keep her locked in the house until morning—then release her.

When daylight came, the entire neighborhood was on alert. Before Misty was released, each home in her route was notified. When Misty was seen, a call to Mrs. Crail was made. Everyone was cooperating. This was a united effort to solve a mystery. Even the Wakefields, who had just returned from a week's vacation, participated. Marna watched from our windows.

Misty had no reason to be nervous, for she would never be aware that every move she made would be monitored. Down the fence she came, then onto the barbecue and into our neighbor's yard. She was traced across that yard over a storage shed roof and into the yard on the other side. Finally she disappeared into the Wakefield garage. The Wakefields saw her enter the garage and waited ten to fifteen minutes. She never ventured out. Misty's kittens must be there! Mrs. Crail was called.

The Wakefields were asked to close their garage door so Misty could not get out. Both the Crails, Marna and I, and the Wakefields set about trying to find Misty and her family. We jointly searched the garage—no results. We searched again—still no results. The search became more intense. I reached into a partially opened box and heard a growl. I quickly removed my hand in order to protect my fingers and then notified the search team of my findings.

I carefully lifted the box with its contents from the storage shelf and handed it to the Crails. They gently opened the box and there was Misty taking care of four hungry kittens.

Misty had been locked up with her kittens for the better part of a week while the Wakefields had been away on vacation. Misty was very thin and her body reserves had been severely depleted due to her nursing. The kittens were almost skin and bone but surprisingly active. The four kittens and momma cat were transferred to a new box that had a clean towel in the bottom. Misty now seemed content and very trusting. She had been reunited with both her feline family and her human family.

Misty in her dehydrated state obviously could not supply the necessary volume of milk required to nurture her growing family. The Crails wanted to do what was best and they turned to me for a suggestion. All five needed some supportive treatment in the way of nutrition to give them a boost to get over the critical stage. The Crails followed me to the Torrance hospital.

I checked each of the kittens over and Misty as well. Misty did not object and must have realized that I was trying to help. Each kitten was given several milliliters of a five-percent solution of saline and dextrose subcutaneously in the napes of their necks. Misty was given fifty milliliters of the same solution. Liquid vitamins were dispensed and a proper diet for Misty was recommended.

Misty's progeny grew into a healthy family. Finally the day came for the Crails to find homes for the four new arrivals. They were quite capable of surviving on their own. I was out in the yard one Saturday afternoon when Ann walked down with one of the kittens and said it was a special gift for me. The boys were with me and thought it was a great idea. Faux Pas thought differently so we had to decline the very generous offer. Marna and I were both pleased with the decision but the boys were out of sorts for a few days.

We finally thought of a way to discourage their idea of acquiring another pet. We explained to the boys that we did not wish to hurt Faux Pas's feelings. If we acquired another cat, she might run away because she might think that we did not love her anymore. This apparently satisfied the three boys and took some of the pressure off both Marna and me. The Crails let it be known in the neighborhood that I was not willing to accept compensation of any kind for the services I had rendered.

I went inside the house to pour myself a glass of iced tea when the phone rang. The San Pedro hospital was connected via the operator. Soon I was on my way to see the Milne family and their Doberman, Charlie, who had broken his nose. There was no question about the complaint, for when I saw Charlie, the nose injury was very evident. It appeared that he might be able to sniff around a corner without exposing his body. Charlie's nose was at a right angle to the rest of his face.

Mrs. Milne had gone to the market and taken her two children with her. Charlie had also gone along for the ride. As she got out of the car at the market, she told her children, "Don't let Charlie out!" This meant to shut the door quickly to them. They slammed the car door. Charlie cried in pain. Mom and her kids went grocery shopping.

When they returned to the car, blood was everywhere. Charlie had a broken nose and had sneezed considerable blood—it was located on the seats, the dashboard, and the windows. Charlie's nose was also "out of joint."

Mrs. Milne took the family home, unloaded the groceries, and put Charlie in the backyard. She then called her husband who was working late. He was not available so she left a message. Then she returned to the car and cleaned it up. Finally her husband called back and suggested that she take the dog to a veterinarian. Charlie was still sneezing intermittently so blood again decorated the seat, dashboard, and the windows.

I asked Mrs. Milne to bring her dog into the treatment room and had her children stay in the reception room. Charlie objected when I first touched his nose and then anytime after that when he even thought I may be reaching for his nose, he would turn his head. Mrs. Milne was not strong enough to restrain her dog properly so a sedative of surital was administered in the vein with her assistance.

Mrs. Milne retired to the front room with her daughters while I tried to realign Charlie's nose. Every time I placed it in the proper location and then laid his head down on the table, the nose would snap back into its adverse position. This plan was not working and a more sophisticated method needed to be implemented. This was going to take more time than I had originally anticipated so I stepped out to my car and brought in the gas anesthetic machine and connected my patient to it.

Now I did not need to rush. I still needed to figure out how to resolve the problem. I finally took a curved aluminum meta-splint and cut the foot support off of it. The curved portion of the splint was bent to conform to the bridge of Charlie's nose. I cut off the length of the splint so that it only extended to the very tip of his nose. The fit was perfect. The problem I now faced was how to secure it so that it remained in place and did the job that was required of it. Two small holes were drilled in each corner of the splint. The underside of the splint was now padded and placed over the Doberman's nose. Stainless steel wires were used to hold the splint in place. One wire was placed through his lip tissue and behind his canine teeth and then secured in place. The second wire was passed through his facial tissue and secured across his hard palate. Both wires were tied snugly so they would not hurt but likely only annoy Charlie. The splint could not move forward or backward, nor could it tilt or move laterally.

I asked Mrs. Milne and the girls to come in and showed them Charlie's nose protector and explained how he may react to this inconvenience at home. They helped me put him in a cage. I wanted to keep their dog under observation to see how he would react to the apparatus when he was awake and on his feet. I told them I would call later, and then they could come down and take their dog home.

I returned to the hospital later that night. Charlie was on his feet with his nose poked through the bars on his cage. A distinct klunk was heard every time his metal nose splint hit the cage bars. This could be a problem. I was afraid that he would be bumping his nose at home also. He made no attempt to wipe the splint from his nose with his front feet—probably because his nose was too sore. More protection appeared to be essential.

I called the owners and asked them to come and pick up Charlie. Mr. Milne had come home and he accompanied his wife and children to pick up their dog. I dispensed an Elizabethan collar which fits in a curved manner around the neck. It attached to Charlie's regular collar so it would stay in place, and because it was cone-shaped and extended past his nose, Charlie couldn't reach his nose with any of his feet.

He was quite a sight when all the Milnes saw him. They stood there and shook their heads. I demonstrated how easy it was to take the collar off and put it on again. They would have to perform this procedure for he could not eat or drink with the collar in its current position. Also, with the wires across his maxilla, he was to eat only canned food until the splint was removed.

The collar as well as the splint were to remain in place for three to four days. At that time they were to call and make an appointment with the hospital for a checkup. If anything came loose or did not look right, they were to call right away. Mrs. Milne said that her husband graciously cleaned up the car the second time. They both wondered if the car would be messed up again on the way home. The hemorrhaging had stopped, but I sent a towel with them to hold over the front of his collar if he started sneezing again. In any case, they were to discuss any problems with the doctor when the follow-up visit was made. Charlie was still slightly groggy, so Mr. Milne carried him out to the car.

—42—

A Late Night Bath

I was just getting ready for bed when the phone rang. The operator connected me to the Boyces on the phone. The Boyces were expressing considerable concern regarding Dolph, their springer spaniel. Dolph had several dark tumors over his body. Most of these tumors appeared to be in the dorsal neck area. "Could they be these melanomas that we occasionally hear about?" was their primary question.

We conversed for several minutes. The Boyces related that they lived in El Segundo but had just returned from the San Bernardino Mountains where they had leased a mountain cabin for a week. On the way home one of their children had discovered one of these tumors on Dolph's neck. A more thorough investigation revealed that several of them were present on his body. These "melanomas" had probably been there unnoticed for some time, for two or three of them were very large. I started putting all of this information together—longhaired dog, mountains, dark growths, and pendulous in size. I suggested that we might be talking about ticks.

Mrs. Boyce asked, "Are they dangerous?"

"Not particularly unless they transmit Lyme disease, which is rather unlikely."

"Can they be removed?"

"Yes, they can."

I proceeded to discuss several methods of removal. It became apparent that they had no intention of even touching them. Finally she asked if I could meet them at the hospital.

177

When all of us—Mom, Dad, two boys, and myself got into the exam room, I asked them to put Dolph on the table. They looked at one another and then looked at me. I got the message—no one wanted to touch Dolph. I bent over and placed him on the table. No one desired to hold him during my examination either. I suggested that if they held him by the collar, the ticks would not jump off and infest them. They agreed to restrain him in that manner.

I parted Dolph's coat and noticed a large tick. Several more were also found. The Boyces cringed when I pointed them out and they could see the ticks more closely. Mrs. Boyce asked if they could leave Dolph in my care and pick him up after work the following day. This was an ideal proposal. I said good night. I then carried Dolph into the grooming room and secured him in the bathtub.

I carefully went over his entire body and found several more ticks. I made up a solution of alcohol and a concentrated tick spray. Then with an eye dropper, I placed several drops on each exposed tick. Gradually they released their grip on Dolph's skin and I placed them in a beaker that became my collection receptacle.

I lathered Dolph up with a flea and tick shampoo and allowed the suds to stand for forty-five minutes. Although I had thoroughly inspected him, I found two more ticks that I had missed. Several places on the skin where the ticks had attached themselves were badly inflamed. I gave him injections of a steroid, vetalog, and an antibiotic, chloromycetin, to relieve and protect him as well. I toweled him down as best I could and then introduced him to the drying cage. The heater and the fan were turned on and the timer was set for forty minutes.

By the time I had finished cleaning up the mess around the tub and the examination room, the timer bell rang. I removed Dolph from the dryer cage and located him in a comfortable cage in the kennels. After I had fed him and filled his water dish, I was on my way home.

Just before midnight I responded to a call on the Hermosa hospital line. It involved their cat that the owners, the Harolds, found crying on their front porch. Linus was very weak and could not walk, let alone move at all. How she ever had the strength to get to the front porch amazed the Harolds. We met at the hospital twenty minutes later.

Linus was almost dead when she was placed on the exam table. I was able to easily pass an endotracheal tube and connect her to the oxygen machine. I took an x-ray of her abdomen and rear quarters. She had a fracture of the proximal third of her left femur. Also, there was a density in her abdomen that indicated the presence of fluid. An abdominal tap revealed considerable frank blood so I was very aware of a splenic rupture. Surgery was necessary before she bled to death internally.

Fortunately there was a donor cat present in the ward so I obtained sixty milliliters of blood for the transfusion and went to work establishing an intravenous drip. A ventral midline incision enabled me to expose the contents of her abdominal cavity. The ruptured spleen was immediately clamped off and then the vessels were ligated. When all the vessels were securely tied, the vessels were then cut between the ligations and the spleen was removed from her body. The splenectomy had been completed. The abdomen was lavaged with isotonic saline to rinse it out and to rid it of any clotted blood. The incision line along her belly was then closed.

Linus was doing much better than when I first saw her. She was exhibiting good color and although she had lost considerable blood, it appeared to have been reasonably replaced with the transfusion. The transfusion had been completed so the bottle was disconnected and a liter of saline and dextrose was set up in its place at the rate of one drop every four seconds. Linus seemed to be improving by the minute—a very good sign.

It was not my intention to consider any repair work on the fractured leg that evening, but Linus had shown enough improvement to encourage me to try while she was still under the anesthetic. I clipped the leg over the fracture site that I had located by palpation. The radiograph had indicated it was a clean transverse fracture about two inches distal to the femoral trochanter. I decided to attempt a closed reduction of the femur. (No major incision is required that is any larger than the diameter of the intramedulary pin. All manipulation and alignment is accomplished by palpation.)

The stainless steel pin was put through the skin into the distal end of the proximal portion of the femur. The pin was then drilled through the femoral trochanter so that the distal tip of the pin was now even with the fracture site (retrograde procedure). Now the two portions of the fractured bone were aligned and the pin was threaded down through the center of the distal portion of the fracture until it met opposition. The pin had threads on it and it was then rotated until it was securely held fast in the distal portion of the femur. The extra portion of the pin that protruded out of the skin in the hip area was cut off so it did not interfere.

Partway through the fracture correction, I had turned off the anesthetic machine and just allowed the oxygen to flow. Linus still showed a nice pink color in both her mouth and the conjunctiva of her eyes. When I deflected the eyelid to check her eye, she blinked—the anesthetic was beginning to wear off.

It was time to call the owners. I had sent them home earlier and promised to call when I got out of surgery. The first remark I heard after I had identified myself was, "Did she die?" I brought them up-to-date and told the Harolds that Linus was doing so well that I had fixed the fracture of the leg also. Their boys were up waiting for my call and each one of them had to personally hear my encouraging remarks about their cat, Linus.

It was past two in the morning when all was cleaned up. I had no intention of waiting for the autoclave to sterilize the surgery pack so I left a note for the morning staff to do that for me.

I checked Linus again a little after seven in the morning on the way to my day's work. She seemed to be more annoyed with the pinned leg than anything else. She was still too weak to stand but she was able to hold her head up and watch me as I walked by.

It was very likely that she was hit by a car and had been able to reach the front porch of her home before she lost so much blood that she was weak. At least she had been strong enough to meow at the front door for help.

43

A JUNKYARD

I was going through the day's mail when the phone next to me rang. The operator said that a Mr. Dennison on the Hermosa line wished to talk to me about his dog. I was connected to the client.

"Hey, Doc, Riley's got the same problem again."

"What problem is that, Mr. Dennison?" I asked.

"You know, all that strange stuff he swallows."

"Please refresh me; I don't recall the case."

"Come on, Doc, you've done surgery on my Irish setter twice before."

"I am the emergency doctor covering for the Hermosa hospital—not your regular veterinarian."

"Sorry, Doc, I didn't catch your name."

"That's okay, but what is the problem?"

"Riley chews up and eats anything he can get into his mouth—rocks, plastic, avocado seeds—only to mention a few. He has had surgery on his stomach twice to empty its contents."

"How is he acting now?" I asked.

"Well, he may have swallowed something heavy this time. He has a potbelly that swings back and fourth like a pendulum. He is trying to vomit the stuff up. He stands there with his front legs bent slightly with his head down trying to bring that junk up, but nothing happens."

"Sounds like a case of pica (consuming nonedible objects) to me," I remarked.

181

"Yeah, I think that is what the other vet called it. He's worse than ever before and needs to have surgery, I think."

"Can you meet me at the Hermosa hospital in forty-five minutes?" I asked.

"I'll be there before you, Doc, and thanks for seeing me."

I rearranged my mail into two piles—what I had seen and what needed to be seen. I gave Marna a kiss and headed toward the coast. Mr. Dennison was waiting with Riley. He had given me a perfect description of Riley's current attitude. Riley was gagging and the results were negative. We went into the treatment room and laid Riley on his side and then took one view of his abdomen. We looked at the radiograph together and I was amazed at what I saw. Mr. Dennison said, "It looks like a junk yard!"

I rolled in the anesthetic machine from my car and with the help from my client, Riley was sedated and connected. He was now under anesthetic. Mr. Dennison decided to wait while I was in surgery so I prepared Riley and soon I was standing by the surgery table ready to start.

I excised the abdominal wall and exposed the stomach. Two very evident scars were visible. My next step was to add another incision line adjacent to the previous two. When this was done, I retracted the walls of the stomach, which were very thick due to the abuse of the foreign objects rubbing against them. Mr. Dennison was right—it did look like a junkyard.

A rock about the size of a ping-pong ball was removed first. I found several others that were slightly smaller. A piece of brick and two or three pieces of hard plastic were located and removed. Some unidentifiable small pieces of metal, and lastly, a child's small metal car about two inches long were placed on the mayo tray. There was considerable "gravel" that had settled against the lower wall of the stomach. Some of the gravel was as large as small pebbles. In all, about two cups of this matter were also removed.

The stomach was rinsed out several times to insure that all the debris was removed. I then retraced my steps by closing the stomach and then the abdominal wall. I securely wrapped Riley's abdomen with a roller bandage and some tape to insure that he would not damage the suture line if he tried to wretch again.

I disconnected Riley from all the apparatus and put him into the recovery room. I replaced the IV saline solution that I had started prior to surgery. I collected all of the debris in a large canine feeding dish and took it out and showed it to Mr. Dennison. He said, "That's about normal."

I escorted Mr. Dennison back to the recovery room to take a peek at Riley. His dog was resting well. He bent over and gave the dog a pat and we headed for the front of the hospital. He said, "I have one question to ask you, Doc. Why did you take a picture of his stomach when you already knew all that stuff was in his stomach?" I said, "I wanted to be certain that none of it was blocking his intestinal tract. If there was a blockage there, I needed to be prepared to do that surgery as well."

"Can't you confine Riley to keep him from this habit?" I asked.

"The only answer to that would be a concrete run surrounded by a cyclone fence," he said. "We tried that and he starts barking and disturbs the neighbors. We are between a rock and a hard place—excuse the expression."

I told him that somewhere I had read an article that when pets eat rocks, stones, bricks, and the like that it may be an indication of a craving for salt. "Why not try salting his food lightly and see if it helps," I said.

"It's worth a try, Doc," was his answer.

Mr. Dennison thanked me and we shook hands. We each headed in different directions. I never heard whether my salt suggestion improved the pica problem.

I got home and had just started to go through the rest of the unopened mail when I was again interrupted by Ma Bell. This emergency call also was from the Hermosa hospital. I must have just missed the case, for the operator told me that they were calling from a telephone adjacent to the hospital. I was connected to Mr. Quincy, but it was a very poor connection. I finally asked the operator to act as an interpreter and relay the messages back and forth for both of us.

The Quincys' dog had just hit a car. It made no sense to me. I felt that something had not been transmitted properly in the relayed message. I asked the operator to tell the Quincys that I would be there at the hospital in half an hour.

When I arrived, the Quincys got out of their car and brought in a small Dauchshund. She had fallen two floors. I checked her over and she appeared to be in pretty good shape. Ruby was sore in a few places and walked gingerly when we put her on the floor, but otherwise I gave her a clean bill of health. I remarked that the operator told me that this was a car accident case. "In fact," I said, "I really misunderstood her, for I thought she said that the dog had hit the car."

The Quincys laughed and said, "That's exactly what happened. It was a hot day and we had our sliding glass door and screen open while we played ball with Ruby. We were throwing the ball from the living room out on the balcony for Ruby to retrieve. We had done this numerous times but on the last toss, she slipped and slid under the railing and fell two stories. We rushed to the railing and looked down. There was Ruby lying on top of a convertible that was parked below. We rushed down to her and found that she was alive, but badly shaken up. We gathered her up and headed here and called you from next door. While we were waiting for you to arrive she started perking up. We were so distraught that we used poor judgement—we should have called you before we left home."

I suggested that the Quincys stop at a drugstore and purchase some baby aspirin. I instructed them to give her half a tablet three times daily for stiffness and soreness, and feed her a soft diet for a day or two. The most important thing was to watch her very carefully for any new symptoms, and then to call the hospital if any were noted.

When I got home, Marna told me that she had tried to reach me before I had left but there was no answer. I returned the call to the San Pedro exchange and got the Allisons' phone number and returned the call directly. Their cat, Dené, had been spayed two days ago and she had chewed out a couple of sutures. The Allisons were concerned and wanted me to see Dené to see if everything was okay.

We met at the hospital. Dené was about a ten-pound calico and a jewel to work with. The midline suture row was fine—all she had to do was to leave it alone. I placed a couple of gauze sponges over the suture line and then gave her a body wrap with some elastic tape. She tolerated this procedure very well.

The Allisons informed me that Dené retrieves. I said that I had never seen a cat retrieve. They asked for a sheet of paper and I located one. They then tore it in half and wadded up one half and threw it over on my counter where the supply bottles and thermometer were kept. Dené jumped from the exam table three feet to the counter, picked up the wad of paper, and jumped back. Two more times this was done. Dené appeared proud of her efforts and she was eager to demonstrate her ability.

"Does she know any other tricks?" I asked.

"No tricks, but she is potty trained."

"Potty trained?" I asked.

"Yes" was the answer, "but she only performs when nature calls."

"Come on now, do you really expect me to believe that?" I asked.

Mr. Allison said, "Honey, do you have that photo with you?"

I was handed a photograph of Dené sitting astride the toilet with her tail held up out of the way obviously using the facility in the manner it was intended. Mr. Allison then added that they had to remember to leave the lid up for Dené to perform properly. They could be gone a week—all they had to do was to leave food for her in the automatic cat feeder and leave the toilet lid up. I just shook my head in disbelief.

Later that night, another call came in. Mr. Wexler had a Rhodesian Ridgeback with an angry-looking growth between the toes on one of its rear feet. He wanted me to take a look at it that night because they were going to be on a business trip for several days. I suggested that it could probably wait, but they insisted on having the foot examined that night.

The Palos Verdes hospital was now my destination. The Wexlers arrived with Rhody—a very descriptive name for their dog. We lifted her together and laid her on her side on the examination table. The growth did have the appearance of a melanoma. I did not recommend midnight surgery. The doctor in the morning could do the surgery and then send out a tissue sample. He might even suggest radiation if it was malignant.

Rhody was left for the next day. The Wexlers would call from their destination and talk to the attending doctor. We left the hospital together. Mr. Wexler said, "My neighbor is a physician and he was concerned that the growth was a melanoma too. He thought that it should be checked as soon as possible."

At the next local veterinary meeting, I sat near the veterinarian that did the surgery on Rhody. He said the pathology sample confirmed it was a melanoma. Rhody had already seen a radiologist for treatment but he did not know how effective the radiation treatments had been.

—44—

RED WARNING STARS

I always enjoyed barbecuing. It was my opportunity to have my quiet time. The boys were playing in the backyard. Allen was attempting to organize them in some fashion to play a game, but George and Albert showed no interest in his plans, so Allen gave up and came over to watch me. That evening I was barbecuing ribs, a favorite of the whole family—including Greta who was sitting attentively nearby watching my every move.

Allen wanted to know if he could help me, so I let him turn the rack of ribs. Marna came out and Allen said, "I'm cooking the meat tonight!" He was doing a fine job and my supervision was not needed. Marna came out again and said that dinner was almost ready and asked when Allen and I would be finished cooking.

Just then our neighbor who lived two doors down the street came bursting into the yard with Faux Pas cradled in her arms and holding her snugly so she could not escape. Her dog, Sam, had just gotten hold of her and she was badly injured. Faux Pas spent considerable time investigating the entire neighborhood. Sam was confined to his backyard—most of the time. This evening, however, Sam was out and saw our cat. Faux Pas saw Sam and headed for the nearest tree and sought protection on a limb five feet or so high. She thought that she was safe, but Sam jumped and pulled her out of the tree and likely would have killed her if Sue had not witnessed the event and intervened before Sam had completed his task.

Sue had seen what was happening from her kitchen window and ran outside to save our cat. She had to kick Sam off and then she picked up Faux Pas to keep Sam from getting to her again. She then brought Faux Pas to us. Sue was really scratched up on her face and arms by Faux Pas who had been fighting for her life. She was wild with excitement and her adrenalin was really flowing. Marna went into action. She grabbed a bath towel and smothered our cat in it and then handed the bundle to George. Marna then helped Sue treat her wounds. In the meantime, I asked Allen to finish cooking the ribs. George and I headed for the car. George turned and shouted to Allen, "Save some ribs for us!"

When we got to the hospital, I unwrapped Faux Pas for the first time to inspect her injuries. Most of the damage seemed to be centered on her right rear leg. It definitely was broken, and it was marked by several bite wounds. This was the leg that Sam had grabbed when he pulled her out of the tree.

I took an x-ray. The femur was shattered and several bone fragments were evident around this spiral fracture. George brought in the anesthetic machine and then held Faux Pas while I sedated her and connected the machine. I then prepared for orthopedic surgery with George as my assistant.

It was a complicated fracture as the femur had been splintered longitudinally and several significant pieces of bone were more or less floating in the trauma area. An intramedulary pin was positioned in both ends of the bone. Next the fragments had to be wired in their proper places. Three wire ties were used to hold the pieces correctly around the pin. Two small chips were removed so that they would not damage any surrounding vessels or nerves. Fortunately very little bleeding had occurred because the vessels had not been directly involved. I closed the skin and fashioned a traction splint for the leg so that the splintered pieces of bone would not override each other once she started moving about. The splint would also prevent rotation of the limb enabling the leg to heal in proper alignment.

George followed me into the recovery ward and put Faux Pas in a cage that he had padded and prepared for her. George kept asking, "Will Faux Pas be okay?" I assured him that healing would take place, but that it would take a long time. He wanted to stay in the ward and comfort her while I cleaned up surgery and sterilized the orthopedic pack.

It was a quiet ride home. George had little to say and sat there looking out the car window. I broke the silence by asking him if he thought Allen had saved some ribs for us. He looked at me and quietly said, "I hope so."

Marna had seen to it that some dinner was saved for both George and me. Allen had done a marvelous job barbecuing the ribs, and I considered assigning him a permanent job. We enjoyed our delayed feast. Marna had saved all of the rib bones for George to give to Greta. He was so busy handing out bones to Greta that he forgot momentarily about Faux Pas and her problem. He came back into the house and announced to his brothers that he had saved some of the rib bones for them to give to Greta at a later time.

We all retired to the family room and George was busy describing to everyone how surgery had been done and what his role as assistant had been. The room had a solemn atmosphere and George had the floor to himself without any interruptions—except for the phone that rang.

The operator connected me to the client. The Newsomes had a dog with very fetid breath. Wherever Fang licked them, a terrible odor remained. They had to wash their hands, arms, or face depending on what portion of their anatomy came in contact with his tongue.

The Newsomes arrived at the Lawndale Hospital with Fang, their malamute. Fang was a walking cesspool, for as soon as he entered the hospital the reception room reeked of his problem.

It was impossible to look in his mouth because he was in considerable pain. The Newsomes also observed that Fang ate his canned food more readily than the dry food that required some chewing before he swallowed it. Mr. Newsome placed Fang on the examination table. I reached for his mouth to take a look. That was a mistake! He turned his head quickly and bit my left hand. I knew his mouth was sore. I had no intention of opening his mouth—I only had intended to roll up his lip and take a peek. I now had a two-inch gash from the back of my left hand to my thumb. My hand was beginning to throb. I excused myself and bandaged my hand in the treatment room. While I was in the back of the hospital, I filled a syringe with a sedative solution and returned to the exam room.

I approached Fang more cautiously this time. Mr. Newsome was asked to hold his head tightly and put his other hand around Fang's body so he would hold still enough for me to find a vein and administer the sedation solution. Soon Fang was reclining on the table completely under my control. Both of the Newsomes apologized for their dog's behavior and then repeated the apology when they noticed blood seeping through the bandage on my hand. Fortunately it was my left hand that had been injured, for I was not impeded too much being right-handed.

I opened Fang's mouth and put in an oral speculum. I now witnessed a mouth that was in need of considerable dental work. About this time, the fetid odor that they described became even more evident to me. One molar was abscessed and four others were loose. The only thing that was holding the molars in place was a thick layer of tartar that had bridged across the teeth. All of this was observed on the right mandibular arcade—the rest of the mouth was almost in the same condition. I asked the Newsomes if this ten-year-old dog had ever had dental hygiene. Mr. Newsome said, "I never realized that animals needed that kind of care."

"Fang will need to stay the night. Since he is already sedated, I will take him immediately into surgery and clean up his mouth," I said. "Good" was Mr. Newsome's answer. I then asked the Newsomes to watch Fang for a moment while I brought in my anesthetic machine from the car. I rolled the machine into surgery, came back for Fang, and connected him so he would be under anesthetic. Mr. Newsome said, "I'll call tomorrow and see if I can pick him up on my way home from work."

I locked myself in the hospital and returned to the surgery room. I checked my left hand, which was beginning to throb. The throbbing was even more intense when I put on my surgery gloves and started the dental work. I extracted the abscessed tooth, and when I removed the tartar bridge, four teeth came off with it. A cavitron, a dental hygiene machine, was used to remove the tartar from Fang's mouth. Several more teeth required extraction. His mouth now sparkled. An antibiotic was given. Fang was disconnected from the anesthetic and put into a recovery cage.

I cleaned up surgery and put the dental instruments back into the wet sterilization tray. My hand was really bothering me now. During surgery, I more or less forgot about the bite wound, but now that I had removed the gloves, the throbbing was more intense.

Now that everything was cleaned up and in its place, I could concentrate on my left hand. It was not bleeding very much so I got out the cetacaine anesthetic and sprayed some on. While this was numbing my hand, I located the surgical needle and vetafil suture material. It took eight sutures to close the wound properly. I cleaned up my own surgical mess, took a couple of ampicillin capsules, and headed for home.

About halfway home, I realized that I had been so engrossed with suturing my hand that I had failed to put out any warning flags for the morning staff. I returned to the hospital to perform this task. Little red stars were placed on both Fang's cage card and on his medical record.

My hand was very sore now that the anesthetic was wearing off. It hurt when I grasped the steering wheel. If my right hand had been bitten, I would be driving to the emergency hospital instead of home, for I could not have sutured it myself.

Everyone was in bed asleep when I got home. I slipped into bed quietly without disturbing anyone. In the morning my hand was sore but felt better than the night before. I got a lot of sympathy from the family in the morning. George had a very worthwhile observation: "It's a good thing, Dad, that Fang's case did not come before Faux Pas or you would not have been able to fix her leg." He was probably right.

I reported for work at the Hawthorne hospital in the morning, but had to resign myself from doing any surgery. My hand was too swollen and sore to be comfortable with surgical gloves on. In fact, I was unable to do surgery for the balance of the week.

I checked that morning about the Newsome dog, Fang. The hospital reported that they had no trouble handling him. Fang either did not trust me or his mouth was so sore that he did not want it touched—I prefer to believe the latter.

—45—

A Dog
That Smiled

The call came in just shy of midnight. The Westfalls had a dog that was bleeding from its rear end. Every time it sat down, it left a blood spot. "Would you be so kind as to see our dog this night?" was their request. The operator connected me with the Torrance hospital line; I agreed to meet them at that location at twelve-thirty.

The lights were on and the front door open when the Westfalls arrived with Darby, a forty-pound mixed terrier and shepherd. Darby looked like a movie character. He had a fuzzy beard and a long tail that was constantly in motion. When he was put on the exam table, he rolled back his lips and gave the impression that he was snarling at me. He didn't object when I patted him. In fact, his "snarl" became more pronounced and his tail wagged faster. "What a funny expression," I remarked. "That is the way he smiles at everyone," answered the Westfalls. Darby and I hit it off right from the start.

I turned Darby around and lifted his tail. One large mass was evident and two smaller ones were also present around his anus. The larger one had been abraded and was bleeding. I was looking at several perianal adenomas.

The Westfalls were condominium owners and had no place to keep Darby outside. Inside he was damaging the carpet and furniture wherever and whenever he sat down. "He's had this mass for some time and there has never been a problem until now. I guess it started to bother him so he began scooting. That is when he probably rubbed it raw," added Mrs. Westfall.

I continued my examination and donned some rubber gloves for a rectal exam. The one tumor was so large it was interfering with normal fecal passage. My recommendation was that the large tumor along with the two smaller ones be removed.

Surgery was the unanimous decision. I went to the Mustang to retrieve the anesthetic machine. The Westfalls then held Darby in the examination room while I set up surgery. Then with the owner's assistance, an IV preanesthetic was given and an endotracheal tube passed. Darby was taken into surgery and connected to the gas machine. I bid the Westfalls good night and locked them out as they left. Then I settled down for a night of surgery.

I positioned Darby ventrally on the surgery table. Fortunately Darby had a long tail. The tail was usually in the way when this type of surgery was done, but now I had a tail long enough to deflect it away from the surgical site. I wrapped roller gauze around the tip of the tail and then tied the tail forward near Darby's head. This was one thing I needed to do to keep the surgical field sanitary.

The other thing needed to be done to insure that the surgical area remained clean was to address the problem of possible defecation. I gave a couple of enemas and after all the waste was discharged, I packed the rectum with cotton. To insure that the cotton was not expelled, a purse-string suture was used to close the anus.

The hair was now clipped from the surgical site. I scrubbed his rear end down thoroughly with surgical soap and then painted that area with zepherin. His rear end now looked like that of a red-bottom monkey.

The smaller tumors were carefully dissected out first and the vascularity controlled using an electric cautery. Next, the large tumor, which was much deeper and required more dissection, was removed. The larger vessels were ligated and the smaller vessels cauterized. Two hours later, the last skin sutures were in place and I was removing my gloves.

I removed the purse-string anal suture and replaced the cotton pack in the anus. Next I used six to eight gauze sponges as a pack over the anus and surrounding surgical area. To apply pressure, I untied the tail which had deflected over Darby's back and brought it snug over the anal pack, between his rear legs, against his belly, and tied the roller gauze to his collar. This would apply sufficient pressure to the area and would remain in place long enough to hopefully stop any serious hemorrhaging. If the pack needed to be changed, the morning doctor could do so when he arrived in three to four hours.

I cleaned up surgery, the instruments, and made up the surgical pack. I decided not to sterilize the pack but left a note for the morning staff to do that for me. Wearily I headed for home. It was beginning to rain and I really needed some rest before my regular day shift commenced at the Palos Verdes hospital.

I had just turned out the light on my nightstand when the phone rang. The operator wanted to know if I could answer some questions from a woman who was calling about her dog. She desired to know if a dog that had just lost a tooth was considered an emergency. I agreed to talk to her. A young lady was on the line and was very worried about her five-month-old poodle which had just lost one of its canine teeth. Her dog had been sleeping on her bed and had apparently gotten the tooth caught in the folds of the blanket.

I reassured her that it was likely a baby tooth, a deciduous tooth, and one that was destined to come out anyway in the very near future. No harm was done. She thanked me for taking the time to talk this over at this time of morning and wished me good night—or rather good morning.

At six-thirty in the morning our house was usually stirring. Marna was already up fixing breakfast and making lunches for the boys. I decided to get up too and enjoy some time with my family. A couple of extra cups of coffee helped to energize me for the day ahead. I still had some time on my hands, so I left the house a little early to check on Darby.

Darby heard me enter the hospital and gave me a welcome bark of recognition when I flipped on the light in the recovery room. His vocal greeting was accompanied by a toothy smile. There was no tail wagging since his tail was still tied to his collar and holding the anal pack in place.

As I tried to untie the gauze from his collar, he kept getting his nose in the way and licking my hands. Finally, the knot was untied and the pack fell to the floor of the cage. He was too active to remove the cotton "plug" in his anus, but he cooperated by having a stool and expelling the cotton all by himself.

I spent more time than I had planned, and the hospital was becoming alive with the arrival of the morning staff. I met the doctor entering the front door as I was exiting. We exchanged greetings. He asked if I had been there all night—I said, "Almost!" I did remind him that I neglected to discuss castration with the Westfalls since anal adenomas are influenced by testosterone, and he said he would do so when Darby was discharged.

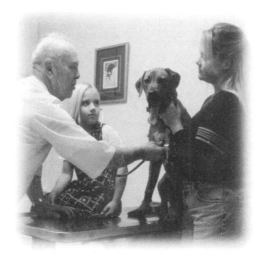

—46—

A Vindictive Client

My first call of the evening was handled over the phone. A woman called and said that she couldn't keep her two dogs apart. One dog was dominant and obese. It would empty its own pan of food and then crowd out the other dog from his. I listened carefully to the complaint and the following question:

"What can I do, Doctor, to keep Charlie from eating Shorty's food?"

"Feed them separately."

"I can't do that."

"Can't you feed one in the garage and the other in the yard?"

"We have only a carport and no fenced yard."

"Where do you feed them?"

"In the kitchen."

"Can't you put a door between them?"

"No!"

"Why?"

"We live in a studio unit and have no doors."

"Most building codes require a door for the bathroom. You do have a door there, don't you?"

"Yes."

"Try feeding one in the bathroom and one in the kitchen. If Shorty doesn't eat all his food, pick it up so Charlie won't eat it."

"That's not easy, for we leave a pan of food out so they can have a noon meal."

"Pets can get along well on two meals a day—morning and night. Control the dietary intake of your animals. Follow the recommendations of quantity on the side of the can or sack of food you feed."

"Are you sure they can get by with only two feedings a day?"

"Yes, I am."

"I'll try it then to see if it works."

The client hung up. From what I could estimate, Shorty had probably been eating one pan full of food daily and Charlie five.

I had just placed the receiver in its cradle when the phone rang again. I almost jumped because it surprised me. The San Pedro operator had been trying to reach me and now she had made contact. Mr. Foster was on the line. He had found his cat dead on the front porch. Mr. Foster wanted me to see his dead cat and do an autopsy. He thought that his neighbor might have poisoned it. I was hesitant about taking this call—it really was not an emergency and could wait until morning. He was very insistent, and after some discussion, I realized that there was no way I would be able to discourage him.

Mr. Foster met me at the hospital in Gardena with his demised cat in a cardboard box. I could feel a lot of fluid in its abdominal cavity and suggested that the cause of death might have been due to trauma. He would not listen to me. I was overruled—an autopsy was imminent.

Mr. Foster insisted on an autopsy because his neighbor had threatened to kill his cat if it did not stop using his flower boxes for its toilet. Poor relations had developed into an almost open conflict. The entire neighborhood had lost its peaceful attitude.

He wanted to wait and discuss my findings. I even told him that nothing of any value might be found and that if tissue samples were taken and sent to the laboratory for analysis, they would cost at least forty dollars each. Even the tissue samples might not reveal anything significant. "That's okay, Doc, go to it!" was his response.

I proceeded with the autopsy. The abdomen was full of blood. The diaphram was ruptured and a large rent in the spleen suggested a traumatic blow of some intensity. I took my gloves off and went out front to relate my findings to Mr. Foster.

"If he was hit that hard, who put him on the front porch?"

"It is likely that he had enough strength to reach the front porch himself before he bled to death," was my response.

"That's hard to believe. I still think he was poisoned."

"It is not likely," I added.

"Look, Doc, if you don't want to do what I requested, let me know and I'll find a vet that will take samples."

"I won't argue with you. I'll collect the needed samples," I said.

I regloved and proceeded. Several tissue samples were taken of the liver, kidneys, and lungs as well as intestinal tissue and its contents. Mr. Foster was sullen when I returned to the reception desk. He paid my fee as well as the three-hundred-dollar deposit for the laboratory work. He handed me four one-hundred dollar-bills and I had to go to the restaurant down the street to make change.

Mr. Foster managed to thank me for my evening's work and said, "I'm going to fix that guy for poisoning my cat if it's the last thing I do." I later found out that all the samples were negative.

When he left, I put his feline in a cadaver bag and cleaned up. It was a shame that he was such a vindictive person. He obviously was a very difficult person to have as a neighbor.

I called Marna and found that I had a call waiting. A client who was planning to ship his dog by air could not find the rabies certificate required by the federal government to verify that his dog had been inoculated.

I had to go right by the Torrance hospital on the way home. I stopped there where his dog's records were and made out a duplicate certificate. I had just completed the form when the client arrived. It was finally time to go home.

— 47 —

KICKED BY
A HORSE

It was afternoon on Saturday when the Waynes called. Their dog, Jeb, had a broken jaw, and they were calling from a phone near the San Pedro hospital. They had gone directly to the hospital when their dog was injured and forgot that the hospital closed early on Saturday.

They lived near a horse trail in the Palos Verdes peninsula. Jeb was a six-month old springer spaniel with a curiosity about all the horses that passed by their yard. He had run out of the yard, and being unacquainted with horses, had approached one of them from the rear only to have the horse kick him in the face. He came running back to the house and the Waynes noticed his injury right away because he could not close his mouth completely.

When I got to the hospital, the Waynes were walking Jeb in the parking lot. Jeb was drooling profusely as he could not swallow the saliva he was generating. Jeb was given a sedative right away so we could position him properly, and then several x-ray views were taken. Two fractures were evident. One was a mandibular symphysis fracture or separation and the other was a fracture of the right mandible.

I discussed with the Waynes the method of correction and the aspects that needed to be considered. Mr. Wayne held Jeb while I went out to the Mustang and brought in the Heidbrink machine. Jeb was connected to the gas anesthetic. I walked to the front door with the clients and locked the door and then went into surgery and set out the

198

necessary instruments and equipment needed.

Jeb was a young dog and young bones heal well. The biggest problem that needed to be addressed was the stabilization of the jaw. The fracture would need to be securely held in place and remain that way for four to five weeks. An intramedullary pin was placed in the mandible and the portion of the pin that extended beyond the mandible was cut off, leaving only about one-fourth inch exposed. The exposed portion was left so that the pin could be recovered when the mandible had healed properly. Now I had to correct the symphysis fracture. This fixation was accomplished by wiring both halves of the mandible securely together. Now all the bones of the jaw were properly positioned. Keeping them there for the necessary period of time would be up to the management of the patient by the Waynes. I disconnected Jeb and placed him in a recovery cage.

One of the biggest problems was keeping the dog from chewing any hard object. This problem was magnified for a pup cutting its adult teeth because puppies love to chew on anything that can fit into their mouths. The recovery plan would have to be worked out between the attending doctor who would discharge Jeb and the Waynes. I anticipated that the wire could be removed in about three weeks and the pin two to three weeks later. No bone chewing was advisable for three months. Upon the pin's removal, the jawbone would be weak for awhile before his jaw could be tested in any manner.

I called the Waynes and gave them the postsurgery report. The surgery pack was put into the autoclave and I sat down with a cup of coffee. I called Marna. No further emergencies were on my current agenda. I was able to enjoy two cups of coffee before the time on the autoclave indicated that sterilization had been completed. I vented the autoclave, and when the pressure was reduced enough, I opened the door so the instruments could cool.

When I had conversed with Marna, she had asked me to stop by the grocery store on the way home to pick up some milk. While there, I decided to get some hot dogs and buns to barbecue. Doing this would give me an opportunity to be outside with the boys. After leaving the store, I remembered that Marna had planned a meat loaf for supper—hopefully she could hold it over for the next day.

When I arrived home, Marna was surprised that I had changed her evening's menu, but she agreed that meat loaf for the next day was acceptable. We finished our supper in the backyard at our picnic table. Allen and I were busily engaged in a conversation when Albert, who had been in the house, kept trying to interrupt us. Finally he had his opportunity—he tugged my sleeve. He burst out with, "Telephone, Daddy!"

The operator connected me with the Philpot family. They had a dog that had just been hit by a motorcycle. Oscar, their German shepherd, had an injured foreleg and was bleeding from his mouth. They wanted to meet me right away at the Redondo Beach hospital. I left immediately.

Both Mr. and Mrs. Philpot brought Oscar into the hospital. We went into the treatment room and my examination commenced. Oscar was still a little dazed from his experience. I could feel the crepitation when I palpated the right scapula. Next an x-ray was taken and a fracture was confirmed. I bound his shoulder tightly to his body and then placed a hobble around the right humerus of the injured leg to the same area on the other leg. This hobble would keep him from moving his leg laterally and causing more damage.

Next I started an intravenous drip of saline and dextrose and added solu-delta-cortef to it to counteract any aspects of shock. His mouth exhibited one space where a tooth had been and two other teeth adjacent to that spot that were very loose. His tongue had been bitten and that accounted for the bloody discharge from his mouth.

Oscar would remain in the hospital the rest of the weekend. On Monday the doctor would evaluate the fracture and plan a course of action to correct the problem. I would monitor Oscar's progress later that night and several times on Sunday to see that he was properly cared for. The Philpots felt Oscar would be in good hands and were comfortable with my recommendations.

As we walked to the front of the hospital, Mr. Philpot related the circumstances of Oscar's injury to me. "Oscar sure caused a lot of activity and excitement in our neighborhood," said Mr. Philpot. "Oscar got hit and was knocked to the side of the road. The motorcyclist lost control of his cycle and it hit the curb. He was thrown up over the handlebars and was injured. The cycle continued for about twenty or so feet and hit the car in our neighbor's driveway. The next door neighbor witnessed the entire event. I quickly checked Oscar over and with the neighbor's help, put him in our car. My wife called you. Before we left, the ambulance was arriving to take care of the cyclist, and when we got to the first cross-street, the tow truck was coming around the corner to, I presume, haul the damaged motorcycle away. I imagine that I will have a lawsuit of some kind over this."

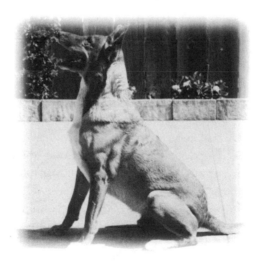

—48—

IMPALED ON
A STAKE

Sometimes clients are so unhappy that they let their emotions get the better of them. I was faced with this problem one night. The operator had passed this phone call along to me because she had refused to talk to the client any longer as he was loud and boisterous.

I could not understand exactly what the problem was. It concerned their male cat, Frisco, and I was talking to a Mr. Kramer. He was very upset, but not at me. He was a pilot and had just returned home to find that his cat had likely been poisoned. There had been a rash of poisonings in the area, and he was almost certain that that was what had happened to Frisco.

Mr. Kramer wanted to bring Frisco to the hospital and have him put to sleep because he could not sit around and watch his cat suffer through a slow demise. We met at the Torrance hospital.

Mrs. Kramer had found their cat on the back door steps and he could not walk. A neighbor had a cat with similar symptoms and it had been diagnosed as being poisoned, so obviously Frisco had gotten a dose of the same poison and would soon die. The neighbor's cat had lived three days before it died. She had felt that nothing could be done, so why waste money by taking him to a veterinarian. Now I began to understand what had infuriated Mr. Kramer—a poisoned neighbor's cat and his wife's failure to take Frisco in for medical attention.

When Frisco was put on the exam table, he would try to walk, but the best he could do was to drag his rear legs around. He could not stand up

202

on his rear quarters. I suspected a thoracic or lumbar fracture of his spinal cord. Mr. Kramer had calmed down a good bit by now, and we agreed that it would be best to look at a radiograph to confirm any action we might have to take.

With a cat, I usually administered the intravenous sedative in the femoral vein of a rear leg. When I touched the leg, I noted that it seemed rather cold. The opposing rear leg was cold too.

I was now suspicious of a vascular problem. With Mr. Kramer's approval I administered a solution into the vascular system that would highlight the arterial supply to the body. An x-ray was taken, and we looked at the film together on the viewer. No spinal fractures were evident. The solution enabled us to trace the arterial supply down the aorta to the bifurcation of the femoral arteries. There it stopped. The rear quarters were void of a blood supply at the junction of the aorta and the arteries that supplied the rear legs. An embolus (clot) had formed and blocked circulation at that location. I paid more attention to the rear legs and this time noted that the skin was leathery to the touch and was very pale in color.

I put Frisco in a cage and returned to the reception room and sat down with Mr. Kramer. We talked over the facts that had been discovered. Mr. Kramer decided to have me euthanize Frisco. He signed the necessary papers and I returned to the rear of the hospital and fulfilled his request.

When I returned to tell Mr. Kramer that the task had been completed, he said, "It was a bigger investment than I had expected, but it is gratifying to know that someone in our neighborhood was not poisoning pets." I remained silent about the actions of his wife. If Frisco had been seen earlier, very likely the clot could have been removed and he would still be alive today. I mentioned that the problem with Frisco was unique and unlikely related to the neighbor's cat's problem.

As it was early evening, Allen decided to go with me on my next emergency. He didn't have to wait long. We had just finished supper and Marna was getting dessert ready. The boys were clearing the table and I was rinsing off the dishes. George answered the phone. "Dad, the emergency operator wants to talk to you!"

The operator said, "I have a Mr. Belanis on the Gardena line. He has already been advised about the emergency fee. May I connect you?" I said,

"Yes." He informed me that his Labrador had a nasty wound on its shoulder. "Smoke has a habit of jumping over the fence in our yard and he must have hurt himself when he landed on the other side. He's bleeding badly."

I instructed him to wrap his dog in a towel and head for the Gardena hospital, and I would leave too, but that it would take me twenty minutes to get there. I stuffed a brownie in my mouth. Allen grabbed two or three and we headed for the door.

Shortly we arrived at the hospital. Mr. Belanis had done a good job of wrapping Smoke in a large beach towel, and his wife had done the driving while he kept the towel in place. He carried his Labrador in and placed him carefully on the treatment table. Smoke could stand on all four feet, but he was not inclined to move about too much.

I removed the towel and it was blood-soaked. Several large clots were visible on the towel. Before I attempted to do any probing, I explained that I needed to have Smoke absolutely still as I did not want to cause any further damage. Allen held Smoke while I administered surital and then Allen brought in the gas anesthetic machine from the car. With his help we entubated Smoke and connected him to the gas anesthetic.

Mrs. Belanis had problems with the sight of blood and was light-headed so her husband took her home and remained there with her. I was to do everything I could do to help Smoke. When finished, I was to call him at home.

I packed the wound on his right shoulder. Allen kept handing me gauze sponges. When the bleeding finally stopped, we carried Smoke in and placed him carefully on the x-ray table. Both a dorsal-ventral view and a lateral view were taken. Considerable debris was noted when I examined the radiograph. I placed a sounding rod as deep as I could into the wound to determine the depth of a solid object and took one more view. A foreign object about three inches long was delineated on the radiograph. Several pieces of the same material also were disbursed in that area.

I was able to locate this unknown object after I had removed the sounding rod. Several attempts were made to grasp it with a large allis forceps. Finally I got a good grip on the large piece and with gentle maneuvering and slow extraction I was soon holding a large foreign body in front of the surgical light. Allen took it and washed it off—he identified it as a piece of wood. Smoke had jumped over the fence and impaled himself on a garden stake.

Smoke had been very fortunate. The wood "spear" had passed behind the scapula and over the brachial plexis and embedded itself deep in the muscles. I tied off several vessels that were still bleeding and removed several fragments of wood. All the gauze pads were carefully counted as they were removed. We waited a few moments to see if any significant hemorrhaging would commence again. When no major flow of blood was noted, the wound was packed with antibiotic powder and the shoulder was bound tightly to the body—first with gauze and then with elastic tape. Antibiotics were given intramuscularly to prevent infection from any contaminates that may have accompanied the wood into the lesion.

Allen had disconnected the anesthetic machine when I started bandaging Smoke's shoulder. Now Smoke was trying to raise his head and inspect the bandage. Allen assisted me in carrying Smoke into the recovery room and placed him in a padded cage that he had earlier prepared. It was a job for both of us to carry an eighty-pound dog through the doorways and place him in a cage.

We started to clean up, but Allen suggested that I call the Belanis family and give them the report. This would save time. I made the return call. Mr. Belanis was pleased and wanted to come right down and see Smoke. I discouraged him because I did not want Smoke to become excited and have the hemorrhaging commence again. He agreed that that made sense.

I was just about to hang up when he said, "I took a flashlight and looked over the fence. Smoke landed on a three-foot-long stake and it must have taken him some effort to get free because several plants were knocked down and the area was a mess. I knocked on my neighbor's door and he turned on his floodlights. We found one broken stake that had lots of blood on it." The neighbor went on to say, "Smoke usually jumps back over the fence, but this time he came out through our yard and wanted in your yard through the side gate. When I went out to let him in, I noticed that he was hurt. I tracked the blood spots to find where he had injured himself."

Mr. Belanis made me feel proud when he said that Allen sure knew what he was doing and would likely follow in my footsteps someday. I asked him to check with the hospital in the morning, for as soon as that doctor arrived, the case would be his responsibility.

Allen suggested that we take a surprise home for his mother and brothers. I agreed and asked him what he had in mind. Without hesitating, he said, "Pie." I stopped at the local restaurant-bakery and gave him some money with the comment, "Pick out whatever you like." He returned with a luscious-looking fresh strawberry pie, and said, "Mom likes this best." I thought that he was very thoughtful.

We sat around the family room and Allen gave a detailed description about the emergency while all of us indulged in the strawberry pie. Albert became a little pale at times and reminded his brother that we shouldn't talk about what Dad does at the office while we were eating. Allen retorted that those rules only apply when we were at the dining room table. Marna and I smiled at each other and just decided to listen to the banter.

—49—
A DIFFICULT BIRTH

My first call of the evening involved a dog with an injured foot. The foot was swollen and Skip would not use it at all—let alone stand on it. I agreed to meet the Winstons at the Redondo Beach hospital. It was almost bedtime for the two youngest boys so I bid them goodnight and told George that I would drill him on his multiplication table in the morning.

The Winstons brought in Skip. His paw was badly swollen but did not appear to be infected. When they related to me the circumstances of the injury, I felt it was that likely that it had been crushed. An x-ray was necessary and I asked Mr. Winston if he could hold Skip and position him so that I would not have to sedate him. He agreed to try. Skip, a brown-and-white-colored cocker spaniel, was very easy to handle. The radiograph revealed two fractures—both of the metacarpals, bones of the right front foot. The swelling was caused by the trauma of the injury.

As the bones were still in alignment, I fashioned a metasplint to protect the foot and securely taped it to the injured paw. A steroid injection was given to reduce the swelling. Care was needed when the foot was taped to allow for sufficient circulation. Then, at the last minute, I decided to give Skip a tranquilizer injection to keep him quiet.

While I was taping the splint to the foot, the Winstons related to me the circumstances of the injury. "We didn't see the accident happen," said Mr. Winston. "I lift weights and have a set-up in the garage for conditioning.

When I got through exercising this evening, I put the bar with its weights still attached back on the stand. At dinner we heard a loud sound, and then heard Skip yelp. Then it was quiet. Later when I went out to the garage, Skip met me at the door with his paw elevated. That is when I noticed that the weights were off the stand where I had placed them. Skip must have knocked them off onto his foot."

Since I had wrapped the swollen foot and knew that the medication would reduce the swelling, I suggested they bring the dog to the hospital the next day for a checkup. The support for the foot would have to be readjusted to fit the smaller paw when the swelling went down. As they were thanking me and asking a few more questions about Skip's aftercare, the phone rang on the hospital's back line. It was Marna. She asked me to contact the answering service of the Palos Verdes hospital about an emergency.

It took me only a minute or two to clean up the area. I then called the exchange. The Carson family had a German shepherd in hard labor. Freeway had been in labor for almost three hours without any results, and they felt that it was long enough. They asked if I would be so kind as to see Freeway as soon as possible.

It would take them about twenty-five minutes to get to the hospital. I was only ten minutes from that location so I was on my way in a rather leisurely fashion. I thought of Allen and how I might need his assistance in the case.

When the Carsons arrived, I did not even have them stop at the front desk. They followed me into the treatment room—all of them—Mom, Dad, sister, and two brothers. Freeway was straining and in full-blown labor. I gloved and checked her digitally. A fetus was across the birth canal.

I suggested that Mrs. Carson and her three children wait in the front room while Mr. Carson remained with me and held Freeway's head. Mrs. Carson instructed her daughter and sons to return to the reception room and look at some magazines or other material. She announced to me, "I'm staying. I'm an OB nurse!" Great, I thought, Mrs. Carson would probably be a more knowledgeable assistant than Allen.

There was no need to give the hormone, oxytocin, to cause Freeway to strain for she was already doing a very efficient job in that respect. What I needed to do was to work between her bearing-down attempts.

The fetus needed to be repelled and then moved to the left since its head was to the right. The fetus also needed to be rotated. If this could be accomplished, all of us could witness a normal delivery. I explained my intentions to Nurse Carson and she agreed with my method of approach.

Finally Freeway eased up a bit on her straining and relaxed enough so that I could push the fetus laterally using digital manipulation for the better part of an inch. Freeway had a large enough pelvis to enable normal delivery if I could only manage to align the fetus properly in the birth canal. Four times she momentarily relaxed and each time I was able to move the fetus slightly to the left. Finally I could identify an ear. One more relaxation and I was able to swing the nose of the pup into the birth canal.

I was certain that Freeway was now completely fatigued by this time, and I was considering giving her a hormone injection to again enable her to assist me. All of a sudden, she gave a gigantic push and the first pup was in my hands. I wiped the amnionic sack from its face, cleared its throat, and gave it a gentle shake—no results. The pup was unable to respond. It had been detached from its mother too long and squeezed too much. It had died of anoxia.

Now the maternity ward came into full action. The second pup arrived and I repeated the procedure. It started breathing so I placed a clamp on its umbilicus to stop any bleeding and handed it to Nurse Carson. I started to tell her what to do, but she said, "I know all about this with babies—here comes another one!"

Four more pups were delivered in the same manner. Nurse Carson was a great help. She put the five viable pups on the floor in the corner of the room. They were squirming around and making all sorts of normal puppy sounds. I removed my gloves. I wanted to give Freeway a clean-out injection to enable her to discharge any retained afterbirth. When I palpated her abdomen two more pups were found to be still retained. A hormone injection was given and Freeway was put into a cage for observation for a few minutes.

I now had time to find a box and line it with towels. The five live pups were put in it and Nurse Carson took it out front to show her daughter and sons.

Freeway started straining again and delivered the last pups without any assistance. Now I had the chance to take a look at all of the seven pups in the box. The pups did not look like any German shepherd puppies that I had ever seen before. They all had shepherd heads. Some had large black spots on them and several had white vest-like streaks on their chests. I asked the Carsons who the sire was. They looked at me and shrugged.

The Carsons had been driving along a freeway about a month and a half ago. Running down beside the center divider was Freeway. "We were in the fast lane and tried to encourage the dog to get off the street before it got hit and killed. That didn't work. Since there was no traffic, my husband pulled over to the left about fifty feet in front of this dog and opened his door. She jumped in across my husband's lap, and then immediately into the backseat. I was petrified and Walt was very concerned. Thankfully our children were not with us. Freeway proceeded to wag her tail and lick our hands. I think she was thanking us.

"We continued home with the idea of having the pound pick her up the next day. The children bonded with her right away and she was very gentle with them. The fur on her neck indicated that she had worn a collar. We advertised in the newspaper trying to find her owners for almost two weeks. We decided to keep her even though we realized about that time that she might be pregnant."

"Doctor, she is a wonderful pet. She gets along well with the family and we plan to keep her. Don't even ask how she got her name." I smiled and could see the affection Freeway had for her human family and the way they felt about her also.

"When the pups get to the 'giving away' age, Doctor, you can have the pick of the litter." I declined and suggested that with Christmas coming up in a couple of months, they should have an easy time finding homes for all seven of the pups.

I thanked Mrs. Carson for her expert assistance and watched from the front door as they left. Before they had pulled out of the parking lot, another car pulled in. They had been told that I was at this hospital and since they lived only a short distance away, they took the chance of catching me on location before I left.

Their poodle, Pepe, had started coughing that morning and when they both got home from work, the coughing was much worse.

I filled out the data that was necessary for the medical record. Pepe was still coughing intermittently. He had a mild temperature and his throat showed considerable irritation. I could not ascertain if something directly caused the irritated throat or if it was secondary to the coughing.

The owners informed me that both of them had missed a few days of work recently with the flu. A sinus congestion and a sore throat had been their symptoms. "Could Pepe have the flu?" I told them that viruses sometimes will transfer to another species—at least that was reasonable to my way of thinking.

I planned to treat Pepe symptomatically. An injection of the antibiotic, ampicillin, and another of the steroid, vetalog, for the irritated throat were given. I prescribed both of these in tablet or capsule form and also dispensed some hycodan for the cough. A honey and water solution was recommended to comfort him and coat his throat. I had some of this mixture on hand and gave him some—he was quiet for awhile.

I made an appointment for two days later at that hospital, but asked the owners to call sometime the next day and give the hospital a progress report. I headed home after cleaning up.

As I turned the corner and progressed down my home street, I noticed that there was still a light on in the family room. I knew that Marna would be up. She had perked some decaf and we chatted as we enjoyed it. George had stayed up as long as possible so that I could help him with his multiplication table, but Marna had substituted for me and drilled him until he became proficient.

—50—

HIT AND RUN

I noted that it was a beautiful fall evening as I headed toward Manhattan Beach and my forthcoming case. The traffic was rather dense as it can be on a Friday with all of the city folks heading somewhere for the weekend. I decided to circumvent the traffic and take an alternate route. I drove through a residential neighborhood where the liquid amber trees were in full color. This broke the monotony of my normal blacktop route. I had left home early which enabled me to take a more casual trip to the hospital.

About halfway down one block, there seemed to be some activity down the street. I slowed down. Several people were in the street watching this gray poodle that was yowling in pain. I got out of the car and asked a bystander what had happened. He told me that the dog had just been hit by a car. The driver had stopped his car, got out, looked around, got back into his car, and departed.

Now this little poodle was sitting on its rump spinning around and yelping. Whenever anyone got close, the dog would pivot on its backside and snap at whoever tried to assist it. No one was very bold, but I didn't blame them since all that was evident was bared teeth and noise.

I asked a bystander to get me a blanket or beach towel and in a matter of minutes one was in my hands. I threw the towel over the dog so it could not see what it was trying to bite. This was finally accomplished after several attempts. I reached down over the poodle and placed a hand on each side of the dog's head. The bystanders became more bold and asked what they could do. I instructed one of them to get my handkerchief out of my hip pocket and tie it around the poodle's mouth when I was ready. Gradually I slid the towel from the dog's head and now could hold its mouth shut by surrounding it with my fingers. My helper was then able to use the kerchief as a muzzle and securely tied it around the poodle's mouth. When this was done, I scooped up the dog and took him to the side of the street. Three cars had stopped and about fifteen people had appeared on the scene.

"Who is the owner?" I asked.

"They live down the street, but won't be home until later," came a response.

At this point, I identified myself as a veterinarian and asked, "Who knows the owner?"

A woman came forward and I told her I was taking the injured pet to the Manhattan Beach hospital. I gave her the address and asked her to inform the owners as soon as possible where their pet was.

The little poodle had calmed down considerably. He did not struggle when I transported him, but his eyes revealed that he was very frightened—they were as large as saucers. When I lifted him to put him into my car, I could feel crepitation in his left rear leg and knew it was broken. Also since he wouldn't stand, I was suspicious of a pelvic injury. I placed him on the floor of my car beside me and headed out as the crowd disbursed.

When I got to the hospital, I gave him a tranquilizer. I removed his collar and then cautiously removed my handkerchief from his mouth and put him into a cage. I now inspected his collar. There was a metal tag hanging from the collar that identified him as Waldo.

The case that I had originally intended to respond to was now on the scene. She was a great big lovable golden retriever that the owners were able to control while I recovered a foxtail from her ear. They were soon on their way and I was back paying attention to my accident case.

Since Waldo had now been identified and the owners would soon be located, I was tempted to take an x-ray while Waldo was still under sedation. I felt that it was appropriate, but could not do so without the owner's permission. I decided to put on a cup of coffee and wait a bit. About that time, the front door swung open and the owners, Mr. and Mrs. Brownell, burst into the hospital.

I escorted them into the ward to see Waldo. Waldo was sleeping as if nothing had happened that evening. Permission was granted to take the necessary x-rays. A cup of coffee was offered to them, but they declined and would just wait in the reception area. Waldo had fractures of both the femur and of the pelvis. I carefully walked the owners through my interpretation of the damage. We rechecked our patient in the ward and he was doing fine.

Mr. Brownell said that he could use a cup of coffee now. But Mrs. Brownell was hungry and said, "Let's step across the street and have a sandwich at the restaurant." I was invited to join them. I obliged. We had hamburgers and coffee and chatted about Waldo. When we finished, we again checked on the patient and he was doing fine.

I told the Brownells that the doctor in the morning would be taking over the case as I was only on duty for emergencies. They asked how the doctor would make the necessary repairs involving the femur and pelvis. I reminded them that the doctor would make the proper decisions as to Waldo's well being. I never liked to tell clients what I would do to correct a pet's problem because they may expect the resident doctor to do it the way I described. This is not fair to the resident veterinarian since he might perceive other problems that we were not aware of now and have to make procedural adjustments.

The Brownells were a delightful couple and thanked me many times for rescuing Waldo from the perils of the street. As I threaded my way home through the traffic, the sky seemed bluer and the trees more vivid in their fall colors. It felt good to be appreciated.

About a week later when I returned to the Manhattan hospital, there was an envelope tacked onto the bulletin board with my name on it. Inside was a gift certificate for dinner for two at a nice local restaurant.

It was accompanied by a very nice note from the Brownells.

—51—

BIG DOG NIGHT

Charles Butler, the father of one of George's friends, called me one night and wanted to discuss his dog's plight with me. He had taken his family and dog camping in the mountains, and one night Ranger had gotten into a fight. He wanted me to look at several of the bite wounds—some were angry and not healing well.

I asked George to accompany me and Chuck brought his son of the same age. When we arrived at the Palos Verdes hospital, the boys immediately paired up and I had George show his friend around the premises. I reminded both of them to be quiet in the ward and recovery areas.

Chuck said that Ranger had gotten into a fight at the perimeter of the campgrounds. When he heard the skirmish, he picked up a sturdy stick to break up the fight. When he got to the battleground, several dogs disappeared into the underbrush. Ranger was in pretty good shape even though he was cut in several places. We attended to his wounds and completed our camping trip.

Chuck said, "When we left the park, we spoke with the officer on duty at the entry station and complained about the dogs that had injured Ranger. We were told that several coyotes were causing problems. They scavenged the campgrounds at night and Ranger probably interrupted their routine. As Ranger is a rottweiler, he was big enough to fend the several coyotes off, and then when I arrived on the scene, they headed for cover. They were more leery of man than dog.

"We bathed Ranger when we got home. It was then that we noticed that several of the bite wounds were infected. Is rabies a problem?"

Ranger had been properly vaccinated, but I recommended that he be confined in the backyard for two weeks—house arrest—just to be safe.

Ranger's wounds needed attention. Fortunately the bath had made all of the lesions more visible. Coyotes are smart predators. They would not face the rottweiler head-to-head. One coyote would distract him and the rest concentrate their attack on his rear quarters. The evidence indicated this had happened—most of the bite wounds were on the rear legs and thighs. Some of the wounds should have been sutured, but now that they were infected that was not a good idea.

An antibiotic powder was puffed into each of the wounds and the adjacent hair was clipped off to prevent it from invaginating into the wound and forming a mat over the lesion. A vacuum was used to remove the loose hair and much of the powder as well. Very little loose hair remained in the wound then. What was there was individually removed. The wounds were debrided and cauterized. Ranger was a great patient. Chuck held him and calmed him down and the rottweiler seemed to realize that I was only trying to help him.

After I cleaned the wounds, I treated them with some more antibiotic powder. The lesions would now have to heal by second intention (that is, not assisted by sutures). An antibiotic of pen-strep was given and capsules of ampicillin dispensed. Ranger needed to be rechecked in three days so I made that entry in the appointment book.

I checked with Marna to see if I had any more emergency calls. There were none, so George and I headed for home. When we walked into the house, I was informed that I had another call at the same hospital that I had just left. I called the service and asked them to call the client and tell them that I would be at the hospital in forty-five minutes. George and I had a late dinner. He remained at home and I left for my return trip to the hospital in Palos Verdes.

It was a "big dog night." When I arrived, the client was walking a large Doberman. Mr. Larkin accompanied me into the hospital and after I obtained the pertinent facts, we proceeded into the exam room. Dillon was put on the exam table and I immediately noticed a large swelling on his left rear leg about midshaft on the tibia. This was the leg he had been favoring.

Dillon had been limping on this leg off and on for two to three months, but now it seemed to be bothering him more. This evening when Mr. Larkin had come home from work, his wife told him that Dillon had been carrying the leg all day and seemed to be in considerable discomfort whenever he tried to use it.

It would be necessary to take an x-ray to assist me in any diagnosis. This was done. Mr. Larkin returned to the front room while I developed the film. When I returned with the radiograph, I told him that it was not good news. There was a large boney proliferation on the tibia that also involved the fibula. My provisional diagnosis was that it appeared to be an osteogenic sarcoma.

This is a very bad type of cancer to have because it is so progressive. We talked about Dillon's future. The only way to remove the cancer if my analysis was correct was to amputate above the lesion. This would not be the end of the problem, for even with radiation treatment, the likelihood of this cancer recurring at another location was very probable. I recommended that we send the film to a veterinary radiologist for an expert opinion. The radiologist would advise us what options we faced.

It was a very unhappy evening for Mr. Larkin—he had to return home and divulge this information to his family. The Larkins had bought Dillon just after they were married. The news of Dillon's future would be heartbreaking for his wife and children to accept.

The Browns called and said that their dog was lying at the back doorstep and "quivering." They feared that Freckles, their Jack Russell terrier, was having an epileptic seizure. She had never had one before and they were afraid to go near her.

I reassured them and said that if they could gather her up in a blanket and get her to the hospital I could see her. I held the line for a few minutes and finally they said that they had gathered her up and would head for the Hermosa Beach hospital.

Freckles was uncovered with care after she was placed on the exam table. She had vomited all over the blanket that was used to carry her in. Little brick-colored pellets were visible. "Your dog may have been poisoned," was my comment.

"Those darn kids in the neighborhood are always teasing her and they probably did it because she barks so much at them when they go by on their way to school," the owners said. I started asking questions. Soon I became aware that snail bait had been applied around the yard to control the snail problem.

(In Southern California there is a constant infestation of snails and the residents continually fight them. In order to cope with this problem, many different products are used—most of them contain metaldehyde. Metaldehyde ingestion results in central nervous system disorders. Especially in the spring and summer, but frequently in the fall months, it was necessary for me to treat these snail bait cases.)

Mrs. Brown was asked to go home and bring back the snail bait box so that the ingredients could be more thoroughly identified. Mr. Brown stayed and helped me while an intravenous solution was established and medication administered. Shortly Mrs. Brown returned with the box that was now empty and had to be recovered from the trash. She was astute enough to scoop up some of the pellets in the yard so I could see the product as well. Metaldehyde had caused the symptoms and the Browns were, in a sense, responsible.

More specific medication was now added to the IV drip set-up and Freckles was moved into the ward and placed in a cage with the IV still intact. Freckles was to stay the night. The frequency of the tremors had decreased slightly and it was comforting for all of us to know that the antidote was beginning to have an effect. Freckles was to remain in my care overnight and if she showed any adverse symptoms whenever I checked on her, I promised to call the Browns.

52 —

A RETIRED K-9

I was just getting ready to leave the Hawthorne hospital for the day when Marna called and asked me to bring something home to barbecue for supper. It sounded like a great idea. I stopped at the grocery store and bought a couple of fryers and a loaf of sourdough French bread. When I got home, I changed into casual clothes then went outside and lit the barbecue.

I was standing there waiting for the grill to heat up and enjoying the evening when Albert came running into the yard and announced that Greta had just hurt herself. The boys had been playing tennis with her— they would hit the ball with the tennis racket and she would retrieve it. The ball had been hit into some ivy down the street and when she brought the ball back, she was limping. As soon as she gave up the ball, she lay down and started licking her front foot. Bloody footprints indicated where she had been.

Greta was reluctant to have me inspect her foot and kept getting her nose in the way to obstruct my view. Finally I was able to locate the injury. It was a deep cut between her toes. One of her digital pads was severely cut. I taped a towel around her foot. I started to turn off the barbecue when I realized that Allen could barbecue for me. I asked George to accompany me and we headed for the Torrance hospital, the closest one to which I had access.

With George's help we sedated Greta and put her on the gas anesthetic machine. Now I could remove the clotted blood and inspect the cut more astutely. It was a deep wound and several digital arteries had been severed. The vessels were clamped off with mosquito forceps, then ligated. Now the surgical field was unobstructed by blood and could easily be sutured.

George again held her paw in position and separated her toes to enable me to close the laceration easily. I bandaged her foot first with roller gauze and then securely with elastic tape. George disconnected her from the anesthetic machine. Together we cleaned up surgery and the treatment room.

Greta was carried out to the car and George sat in the backseat and held her head in his lap as we returned home. She was still out of it when we arrived so we found an old blanket and put her on it in the corner of the garage. Periodically some member of the family checked on her. Allen had finished cooking the chicken and toasting the bread. Just before we sat down to eat, I checked on Greta once more—she was doing fine.

We enjoyed a leisurely meal and were sitting around the table visiting when George thought Greta should be checked again. He came back and announced that she had chewed off the bandage and was now chewing at her foot.

I had brought home some bandage material so I could change the dressing in the morning, but now was the time to use it. Greta was not cooperative but with all the help present, we overcame her resistance. One suture had been removed. There was no need to replace it. I now had a problem to resolve that I frequently had to remind my clients about— protect the bandage and keep the pet from undoing what had surgically been done.

One of the boys located a two-gallon plastic bucket. The other two distracted Greta. A hole was cut in the bottom of the bucket to allow just her head to fit through. Then holes were cut on either side of the bottom and ties were put through the small holes and then attached to her collar. We had fashioned an Elizabethan collar substitute.

Greta could stand but she was unwilling to place her injured foot down. I don't think the lesion bothered her as much as the bandage. She tried to reach her bandaged foot with her mouth. She failed because the plastic bucket impeded her. Finally she glanced up at us with a forlorn look. That was when we all laughed at her. George called her "Bucket Head" and that name stuck with her for almost a week. The teasing ended when the bucket was finally removed. I think that Greta realized we were making fun of her. She appeared ashamed and slunk around the house with her head held down the entire time she was modeling the bucket.

Bucket Head's greatest problem was locating the direction of sounds. If she was called, she would look straight ahead and stand in an alert position. If one of the boys would slip up behind her and pat her on her rump, she would jump in surprise. She was the happiest dog on the block when the bucket protection was finally removed.

I had just hung up after talking to the Bakers about their German shepherd, Kato. Kato had cut himself on the right side of his rib cage and he needed some medical attention.

Mr. Baker brought Kato into the Gardena hospital. Kato was somewhat wet and Mr. Baker explained that his dog had a lot of dirt and leaves stuck to his injured side. The injury had happened sometime during the day. The bleeding had stopped but Kato had lain down with his injured side against the ground to keep the flies away that were annoying him. "I hosed him off to clean him up so I could see what the problem was," volunteered Mr. Baker.

I helped lift Kato onto the exam table and then took a closer look. His injury looked as if he had run too closely by some sharp object. The lesion was about six inches long and not very deep because the ribs had protected the chest area. Three rib bones were clearly exposed with a horizontal cut across each of them.

Mr. Baker wanted to know if I planned to sedate Kato. I told him yes. He then said that his dog was very gentle and I could probably suture the lesion while he held his dog. I was skeptical. However, I told him that I would attempt to do it but if it was impossible, then an anesthetic or sedative would be necessary. He agreed to my proposal.

I puffed some antibiotic powder into the wound. I clipped the hair away about two inches on either side of the laceration. Then I vacuumed off the hair and some of the powder came up with it. Any hair left on the lesion was removed manually. The powder kept most of the hair from sticking to the moist wound and saved a lot of time for me in preparing the injured site for surgery. Next I froze the area with a cetacaine anesthetic spray.

Now was the time to install the sutures. Mr. Baker did a fine job in restraining Kato. Kato became a little restless but he quieted down when spoken to. Kato remained in a standing position while I put in almost twenty sutures. He flinched once in awhile, but he was a perfect patient.

I remarked to Mr. Baker that he had a very trusting and obedient dog. He said that he was a retired police officer and managed Kato, a K-9 member of the force. He said that he had held Kato when he had been cut by glass and also when he was cut by a knife by a suspect he had dragged down. "I was his owner and trainer so when I retired, he retired with me."

He asked if he could demonstrate Kato's ability. I said, "Sure!" He asked for my wallet. I hesitated then produced it. He let Kato smell it and then asked me to hide it somewhere in the hospital within Kato's reach. I carefully wedged it under a wall-mounted exam table in the second examination room and I intentionally walked around the hospital to confuse Kato. When I returned, Mr. Baker said, "Find." We sat down in the reception room. Within ten minutes, Kato arrived with my wallet in his mouth.

I made the entries in the medical record and collected the fees for the service I had just rendered. I got out the appointment book schedule for a suture removal date. Mr. Baker said that he could take them out at home in ten to fourteen days. I replied that that would be fine if healing looked okay.

We stood in the parking lot and visited for a few minutes about police dogs and army guard dogs that I had been acquainted with while I was with the army in Korea. Kato stood like a statue by his side until he said, "Sit." Kato then remained in the sitting position until instructed otherwise.

Kato had been the second dog he had worked with on the police force. The first one was a rottweiler that only responded to German commands. It had been trained in Bavaria and brought to the United States for police purposes.

I had bandaged Kato around his chest in order to secure the gauze pads properly. Kato had paid some attention to the bandage earlier, but when Mr. Baker commanded him to leave it alone, he just forgot about it and went on his merry way. As Kato left, I advised Mr. Baker that the bandage should remain on for at least three days and should be reapplied if he started chewing at the suture line. Mr. Baker smiled and said, "Don't worry."

Before I left, I called Marna to see if she had any messages for me. She told me to call the San Pedro hospital's exchange. The operator connected me to the Gilmores. Their Dalmation, Champ, had a problem that they did not understand. When he walked, a funny clicking sound came from him. When he stood still there was no sound. Recently he was spending a lot of time outside—most of the time near a tree. He was raising his leg constantly. "What might the problem be?" was their question.

"Has he been eating?" I asked.

"Not as well as he usually does," was the response.

"Does he urinate frequently?"

"Yes."

"Does he urinate a lot at one time?"

"I really don't know. Gosh, Doctor, if it wouldn't be too much trouble, could you take a look at him tonight? I have to go out of town the first thing in the morning and will be gone for a week. I don't want to have to burden my wife with Champ's problems."

I explained that there was an after-hours emergency fee. He said, "Fine." We agreed to meet at the San Pedro hospital in about half an hour.

When he brought Champ into the hospital, I could hear the clicking he had described earlier—it sounded like castanets. When he stood still, there was no sound. We put him up on the exam table. I first listened to his chest, and as I moved the stethoscope down to his abdominal area, a distinct grating sound was evident. I jiggled his belly and the clicking sound could be heard across the room. Mr. Gilmore said, "That's the sound my wife and I hear when he walks."

A radiographic view of the bladder was taken and both of us were surprised at not only the quantity of bladder stones we saw, but the immense size of some of them. Bladder surgery needed to be done and I brought in the appointment book to schedule a convenient time within the next day or two. "Why can't you do the surgery now?" he asked. I told him the surgery was necessary but not urgent enough to require it that evening.

Finally he leveled with me. He had to go out of town. His wife was an invalid and was more or less confined to the house. She could take care of the dog at home, but she rarely ventured out. "I would appreciate it if you would do the surgery tonight. I don't want Martha to worry. I would like to leave Champ and go home to be with Martha. Could you call me when you get out of surgery?"

What could I say? What he had related to me was reasonable and I told him that I would oblige. It was a surgery that would be simple to do if I had an assistant, but I was accustomed to working alone. I did, however, need assistance in getting Champ under anesthetic. Mr. Gilmore helped me with that task. Together we got Champ sedated and I brought in the anesthetic machine, connected him, and turned on the gas. I then bade Mr. Gilmore good-bye and assured him I would call later.

I placed a stainless steel pan on the mayo tray next to my instruments to save the evidence. Then I made a ventral midline incision in Champ and extended it enough so I could reflect the pendulous bladder through the incision. Now I was able to make the second incision—one through the thick bladder wall. I retrieved several stones with my forceps and then emptied all of the urine from the bladder in such a manner that none of the urine would spill into the abdominal cavity.

Two very large stones forced me to extend the bladder incision so they could be removed. They made a large noise when they hit the metal pan. Then quite a bit of urinary gravel was exposed and removed. A catheter was passed to insure that the urethra was not blocked by any of the stones. Two rows of sutures were required to close the bladder wall. The bladder was tucked back into the normal position in the Dalmatian's abdomen. Two more rows of sutures were needed to close the skin incision. The surgery was now over so I disconnected the anesthetic machine. A bandage was applied around Champ's midline to protect the incision in case he strained. Two large stones, four medium ones, and over thirty pieces of sizeable gravel had been removed.

I called Mr. Gilmore and gave him a surgical update. He wanted to know how long I would be at the hospital because he wanted to take the stones home this evening and show them to Martha.

I put Champ in the cage and left the urinary catheter that I had inserted in place. The surgery pack was cleaned up first and put into the autoclave to sterilize while I did the rest of the clean up. Mr. Gilmore arrived and I showed him the plunder. He said, "I would have had a hard time convincing Martha about the size of the stones, but she will be a believer when she actually sees them." He asked when Champ could go home. I told him that it would be best for him to work that out with the doctor in the morning.

He thanked me, patted Champ, and left. He planned to call in the morning to see how his dog was doing. I kept one of the stones to send to the laboratory for analysis. This lab work would enable the doctor to prescribe the proper medication to control the acidity of the bladder in order to prevent a possible recurrence.

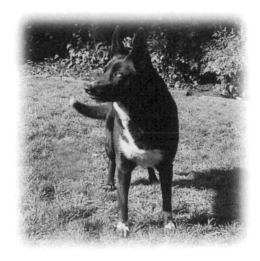

53

HOME REMEDY

The Hansens were connected to me by the operator before I had a chance to ask her what the nature of the call was about. Mr. Hansen said that their cat, El Gato, had a draining wound on his shoulder and the smell of it was overwhelming. El Gato needed to be seen this evening.

I had just finished supper and got ready to go. Marna asked me to put another log on the fire before I left. I obliged. The trip to the Hawthorne hospital was uneventful except for the train crossing. It seemed that there must have been over a hundred cars going by as I patiently waited for the tracks to clear. Then when the last car was almost in sight, the train stopped and started backing up. I just turned off the engine and waited. Finally the road was clear and I was on my way again.

The Hansens were there when I arrived. I explained the circumstances of the delay, and they seemed to understand. El Gato was brought in contained within a cat carrier. The aroma they had described was still present.

We completed the giving and taking of information for the medical record and proceeded into the exam room. Mrs. Hansen removed El Gato from the confines of his cage and then stepped back. I asked one of the Hansens to restrain El Gato while I examined him. Mrs. Hansen volunteered.

El Gato was a longhaired yellow tabby cat with matted fur in many locations over his entire body. His left shoulder was my focal point—his

226

matted coat was moist with pus from a draining abscess. Every time I tried to inspect the wound more closely, he would lay his ears back and glare at me with his big orange eyes. His matted coat also impeded my attempt to make a thorough examination. He did not want to be turned over on his side and the owners were not very interested in holding him due to the odor. I finally suggested that El Gato be sedated now, for it would be necessary for me to have him completely quiet later when I debrided and treated the lesion. I gave him a mixture of acepromazine and vetalar in his muscle and put him into a cage in the ward to wait for the desired effect.

When he was completely relaxed and easy to handle, I took him into treatment and clipped the large stinky mass of hair from his shoulder. It was necessary to trim quite a path of fur off and then I changed to a surgical head on the clippers to cut the fur even more closely around the infected area.

It was definitely a cat bite wound—two very evident punctures were noted. A large patch of skin needed to be debrided as it was no longer viable. After all of the dead tissue was removed, the wound was flushed with a saline solution. The exposed tissue and the fringes of the abscess were swabbed with a tincture of iodine. Vetalog ointment was applied within the lesion and antibiotics were administered.

I returned to the front where the Hansens were waiting to get El Gato's portable cage and I then invited them to come with me to the treatment room to show them how to use the medicine I planned to dispense. They noticed the lingering odor right away when they entered the room—it was not noticeable to me as my senses had adjusted to it.

Mrs. Hansen said, "Maybe we should leave him overnight for a bath." Before the words were hardly out of her mouth, Mr. Hansen asked me if El Gato could be clipped all over now since he was still under sedation. I really did not want to do it at this time of night, but his request was timely. I said that I would remain and do it and told them to call the hospital in the morning. I recommended they take their cage home and wash it with Lysol to control any infectious discharge that may still linger in it.

I began the undesirable task. I almost forgot to change back to the grooming head on the clippers (he would have been trimmed right down to his skin!). Using a comb to hold the mats up, I was able to slip the clippers underneath the mats and remove them. It took a little while and El

Gato was beginning to show some signs of alertness before my job was completed. He looked like a little lion when I was finished. I left the hair on his head intact as well as that on his tail, which I spent some time combing out. I did not know how agreeable he would be in the morning so I decided to put him into the tub to bathe him—it would be a cinch now that he had short hair.

As I was putting him into the bathtub, the phone rang. Marna asked me to call the Torrance hospital's answering service and talk to a Dr. Wells. I asked her to call the service and have them call Dr. Wells and tell him that I would return the call within twenty minutes. I did not want El Gato to wake up so much that I would be unable to handle him.

After El Gato was washed, rinsed, toweled down, and put into the dryer cage, I called Dr. Wells. We made arrangements to meet at the Torrance hospital. As I headed for Torrance, I realized that I knew very little about my forthcoming case.

I arrived before Dr. Wells. He pulled into the parking lot shortly with Arvin, a five-month-old female beagle. Arvin had been vomiting up her meals and fluid about thirty to forty minutes after consuming them. This had been going on since shortly after his wife had wormed her. I checked Arvis over and everything appeared relatively normal except for a soft structure that I could palpate in her abdomen in the vicinity of her intestinal tract. I started asking questions.

"What was Arvin wormed for?"

"She saw some long worms," he said, "but I never saw them because she flushed them down the toilet."

"Where did you get your dog wormed?"

"She wormed Arvin herself with medication she purchased at the pet shop."

"How did they know what product to sell her?"

"She described the worms to them and was told that it sounded like roundworms, especially since Arvin was a young dog."

"When did she worm Arvin?"

"The first time was three days ago."

"You mean she wormed her more that once?"

"Yes. The first time no worms were expelled and she felt that the dosage may have been too small, so she increased the amount and gave it to Arvin the next day—that was two days ago."

"We need to take an x-ray of the gastrointestinal tract," was my next comment.

A series of radiographs were taken after hypopaque, a contrast medium, was given orally. An initial view prior to any medication was first taken and then a series followed at fifteen-minute intervals. When all five films had been processed, I took them to the view screen in the exam room and shared them with Dr. Wells. It was very noticeable where the contrast medium had stopped progressing down the small intestine. The last two views were identical. Arvin had an intestinal block and it was a severe one. Surgery was necessary.

I gave Arvin a preanesthetic injection and then connected him to the metafane gas anesthetic machine. Dr. Wells, a pediatrician, remarked that his diagnostic techniques for the first six months of a child's life were the same as mine. "We both listen, observe, palpate, and then ask a lot of questions of the parents or owners as the case may be. My approach to patients changes and becomes easier once they begin to talk." I thought that was an interesting observation on Dr. Wells's part.

Dr. Wells decided to wait until I had identified the cause of the blockage before he left. I prepared Arvin for surgery and soon I had located the cause of her problem—an intussusception. This occurs when a violent peristolic wave in the bowel overrides a more distal portion. In Arvin, three layers of intestine were now located in one spot. The tissue swells were cutting off circulation. This forms a very complete block and surgical correction is the only way to alleviate the problem. Dr. Wells departed after I informed him the nature of the blockage. He did not dally—he knew that I was in the middle of a complicated surgery.

Each side of the intussusception was clamped off with Doyen's clamps. The damaged portion of the bowel that included the blockage was removed. The exposed ends of the small intestine were united and the intestinal anastomosis was completed. It was almost an hour and a half to complete the surgery before Arvin was placed in a comfortable cage in the recovery ward.

I redid the surgical pack but left it for the morning staff to sterilize because it was past three in the morning and I didn't want to hang around any longer.

Mrs. Wells was trying to correct a problem that existed rather than create one. Sometimes an over-the-counter medication, however, is not utilized in the manner it was intended.

I got home in time to shower and get a couple hours of sleep. I was in slow motion at the hospital the next day and, hopefully, the clients that I saw did not think that I had been out partying too much the night before.

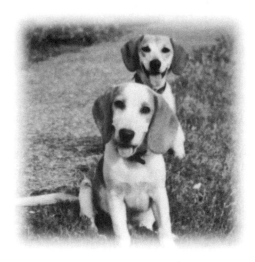

54

CAT GONE CRAZY

Many times I would only have to talk to clients who called. What they needed was assurance that the situation was not an emergency. When I answered the phone this time, the operator said the owner was in a panic. I was connected and the frantic tone of the person on the line dictated my decision. It was hard to ascertain what the problem was. Finally I asked the client to slow down and speak clearly.

Mr. Meade said that his cat had gone crazy and he was scared to have it around his house with small children present. "Mattie was okay this afternoon according to my wife but we found her in the garage after we had dinner and she had gone stark raving mad! She's still out there running around in circles. I am afraid to go near her."

I suggested that he use a thick blanket or spread, throw it over her, and roll Mattie tightly up in the blanket. I would remain on the line until this was accomplished. Five minutes later Mr. Meade picked up the phone and announced that Mattie was safely restrained. All he wanted to do was bring her down to the hospital and have her put to sleep—he was greatly concerned about the safety of his three little children. His wife would drive and he would hold Mattie so she couldn't escape. They would have to bring the three children with them.

We arrived at about the same time and immediately proceeded into the exam room while the children waited in the reception room. Mattie was so wrapped up in the blanket that I could not tell which end was up.

231

Slowly I peeled back the blanket to get a better view of my patient. That was all Mattie needed to escape. Out she tumbled to the floor and one longhaired gray mass of fur was circling the exam room going about fifty miles an hour and bumping into everything in her way.

When Mattie hit the floor, Mrs. Meade made a hasty exit and thankfully closed the door behind her. Mr. Meade got up on the exam table. I was left on the floor with an apparently vicious feline that had gone completely crazy. I grabbed the blanket as Mr. Meade watched from his safe position. On one of her circles around the exam room floor, I was able to flip the blanket over her and scoop her up in a secure manner. Mr. Meade now placed both of his feet back on the floor and said, "Just put her to sleep." He returned to the reception room to comfort his crying wife and children.

There was no way I could administer an intravenous injection to a wild cat all by myself. I had to sedate her before I could locate a vein. It was difficult enough to load a syringe and hold Mattie so that she could not escape again. Finally I was ready. With care this time, I located her rear quarters, then her hip. Now I could place an intramuscular injection through the blanket into her muscle. After several minutes, she had relaxed enough for me to remove the blanket and take a good look. I returned to the front room. Mr. Meade was holding his twins on each knee and Mrs. Meade was involved in comforting the two year old. All were in tears and the parents were actively involved in child care. I explained what had been done so far and that I would return to treatment to complete the task when Mattie was completely still.

Mattie's left rear foot appeared to be stuck in her mouth. Careful inspection revealed a three pronged fish hook. One hook was well embedded in her upper lip and another hook in between the toes of her rear foot. I cut the fish hooks into two pieces in midshaft and then backed out both ends so the barb of the hook was not pulled through tissue. I then stretched her out on the treatment table and that active ball of fur had now become a beautiful grey Persian cat.

I went back out front. Mr. Meade nodded as if to reaffirm that my task was completed. I did not nod back but asked him if he fished a lot. He appeared puzzled. I showed him the fish hook pieces that I had removed from Mattie. I explained that Mattie most likely smelled fish or bait on the hook and in licking or chewing it got one hook caught in her upper lip.

Then in trying to get the hook off her lip, she used her rear foot to scratch it away. Now the interdigital tissue between her toes had become the home of another of the hooks.

I told them that Mattie had not been euthanized. She was safely occupying a cage in recovery, awaiting instructions as to her destiny. The entire family followed me back to see their kitty.

Mr. Meade gave me a hearty handshake. Mrs. Meade awarded me with a thank-you hug. The twins and the little two year old were jumping for joy. Mattie was kept overnight.

As I drove home, I reflected on that unusual evening. It had started out as a night of grief and it ended as one full of joy.

When I passed the local grocery store, I thought that my family would appreciate some ice cream, so I turned the Mustang around and headed back to the store. Chocolate sauce was right next to the ice cream, so of course, it made sense to buy some of that also. When I got home the boys were still up. Marna fixed the dessert and even sliced some bananas to make sundaes. We sat in the family room eating our dessert and I told my family about my evening's experience. Emotional tears first appeared, then as I progressed, tears of joy followed. The boys were already in their pajamas so Marna and I tucked them in. Their bedtime story had just been told and each had a happy face as we kissed them goodnight.

In 1972 it was necessary for me to inform the hospitals where I was taking emergencies that sometime in the future I would have to give up that aspect of my practice career. There was a concern by these hospitals as well as many other South Bay hospitals that something needed to be done to provide emergency service in the area.

A meeting of all the veterinarians in the South Bay was called and from this group five veterinarians were appointed to research the prospect of opening up an emergency animal hospital. I had the privilege of being selected as a representative of the coastal area. It was decided to form a corporation and thirty-five veterinarians became shareholders. The five that were first appointed now became the original board members.

A building was leased in Torrance and then remodeled to the needs of a hospital. The Emergency Pet Clinic of South Bay, Inc. opened its doors in 1974. It was no longer necessary for me to respond to off-hour emergencies.

The emergency clinic was an immediate success. Much of the success was related to the fact that it did only referral work. Cases that were referred to the clinic were returned to the parent hospital when they next opened. Also, the clinic endeavored to provide only emergency services—no routine problems were to be resolved.

The current board consists of veterinarians Teresa Benton, Francis X. Dieter, Robert J. Streeter, Richard J. Sullivan, and myself. With the guidance of Robert Hyman of Diversified Veterinary Management corporation, an accounting firm, and the proper decisions by this board, the clinic in twenty-five years can boast that it has treated over 150,000 emergency cases.

Emergency service means that there is a doctor and trained staff available at all times the clinic is open. The clinic does not compete with daytime practice for it is only open when most of the daytime practices are closed.

My family was elated when the emergency clinic opened. At this time of my life, my role as a husband and father became more traditional. My hours of practice were mostly from eight until five, and I was now home in the evenings, weekends, and holidays with my wife and children.

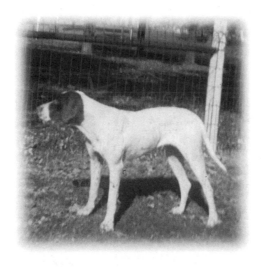

ABOUT THE AUTHOR

George Albert Porter attended the University of California at Davis where he received a bachelor of science in animal husbandry in 1952.

After operating a family farm in Indiana for a year, he was drafted into the army and served in the infantry in Korea for two years. Upon his discharge, he returned to farming and married Marilyn Bradley of Redondo Beach, California, in 1956. In 1957 he decided to return to school, attending Stanford University and graduating from the School of Veterinary Medicine at UCD in 1962.

He opened his own practice, Marina Animal Hospital, in 1970 in Redondo Beach and practiced there until 1990 when he retired as a clinician.

Porter served as president of the Torrance Rotary Club 1968–69. In 1972 he was appointed by his colleagues to be on a committee to explore the possibilities of establishing an emergency pet hospital to serve the many veterinary clinics in the area. This practice, the Emergency Pet Clinic of South Bay, Inc., was an immediate success. Porter has served on the board of directors since its inception.

In 1997 Porter and his wife, Marilyn, moved to Santa Barbara, California, for retirement. While there, he was inspired to compile a series of events from his veterinary career. *PET ER* is the result of his efforts.